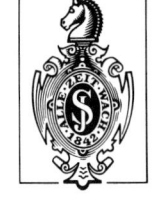

H.J. Deeg H.-G. Klingemann
G.L. Phillips

A Guide to
Bone Marrow Transplantation

Second Revised and Enlarged Edition

Springer-Verlag
Berlin Heidelberg New York
London Paris Tokyo
Hong Kong Barcelona
Budapest

DEEG, H. JOACHIM, M.D.
Clinical Research Division, Fred Hutchinson Cancer Research
Center, 1124 Columbia Street, Seattle WA 98104, USA

KLINGEMANN, HANS-GEORG, M.D.
Department of Medicine, The University of British Columbia
910 West 10th Avenue, Vancouver BC V5Z 4E3, Canada

PHILLIPS, GORDON L., M.D.
Division of Hematology, The University of British Columbia
910 West 10th Avenue, Vancouver, BC V5Z 4E3, Canada

With 12 Figures and 30 Tables

The cover photograph shows a bone marrow biopsy from a patient with severe aplastic anemia before (*top*) and 28 days after (*bottom*) marrow transplantation from an HLA-identical sibling

ISBN 3-540-54831-9 Springer-Verlag Berlin Heidelberg New York
ISBN 0-387-54831-9 Springer-Verlag New York Berlin Heidelberg

Library of Congress Cataloging-in-Publication Data. Deeg, H.J. (Hans Joachim), 1945– A guide to bone marrow transplantation / H.J. Deeg, H.-G. Klingemann, G.L. Phillips.—2nd rev. and enl. ed. p. cm. Includes bibliographical references and index. ISBN 3-540-54831-9 (alk. paper).—ISBN 0-387-54831-9 (alk. paper) 1. Bone marrow—Transplantation. 2. Bone marrow—Transplantation-Complications. I. Klingemann, H.-G. (Hans-Georg), 1949– II. Phillips, G.L. (Gordon L.) III. Title. [DNLM: 1. Bone Marrow Transplantation. WH 380 D311g] RD 123.5.D43 1992 617.4'4—dc20 DNLM/DLC for Library of Congress 92-49684 CIP

This work is subject to copyright. All rights are reserved, whether the whole or part of the material is concerned, specifically the rights of translation, reprinting, reuse of illustrations, recitation, broad-casting, reproduction on microfilms or in other ways, and storage in data banks. Duplication of this publication or parts thereof is only permitted under the provisions of the German Copyright Law of September 9, 1965, in its current version and a copyright fee must always be paid. Violations fall under the prosecution act of the German Copyright Law.

© Springer-Verlag Berlin Heidelberg 1992
Printed in the U.S.A.

The use of registered names, trademarks, etc. in this publication does not imply, even in the absence of a specific statement, that such names are exempt from the relevant protective laws and regulations and therefore free for general use.

Product liability: The publisher can give no guarantee for information about drug dosage and application thereof contained in this book. In every individual case the respective user must check its accuracy by consulting other pharmaceutical literature.

Typesetting: Best-set Typesetter Ltd., Hong Kong
27/3130 –5 4 3 2 1 – Printed on acid-free paper

Preface to the Second Edition

In 1988 we presented our *Guide to Bone Marrow Transplantation*. The reception has been enthusiastic and we have received a flood of critical comments, suggestions and requests to provide an update in due time. Although several books on marrow transplantation have recently been published, their scope and goal have generally been different. Hence, we have decided to prepare a second edition of the *Guide*.

Our aim was to maintain a short, concise text which nevertheless would incorporate changes that have occurred over the past four or five years. We have streamlined the description of pretransplant considerations, by condensing two sections into one (Treatment Planning and Timing of Transplantation). This also facilitated the review of controversial indications for marrow transplantation, for example in patients with acute myelogenous leukemia in first chemotherapy-induced remission. We have updated the chapter dealing with conditioning regimens and have expanded the section on donor selection, in particular in regard to the current level of tissue typing and the identification of unrelated volunteer donors. In the chapter on collection, processing, and infusion of marrow, we have incorporated recent developments, for example, the use of closed systems for marrow harvesting and processing and the use of solid phase separation of stem cells.

In the section dealing with acute transplant-related complications, we have added recent results on graft-versus-host disease prevention, and we have included up-to-date information on the prevention of cytomegalovirus (CMV)-related disease by the use of CMV-negative blood products and treatment with ganciclovir.

We have reworked thoroughly the section on delayed transplant-related complications since a considerable amount of data has accumulated. We have added a section on complications not previously addressed (for example, dental abnormalities) and added a chapter on rehabilitation. Finally, to facilitate retrieval of information, we have generated a small index.

Despite all efforts it is likely that already at the time of publication of this book new results and insights not available at the time of this writing will have changed our approach to certain problems in the field.

We emphasize again that the book was not conceived as a manual on how to do marrow transplants nor as a textbook giving countless statistics. The goal remains that of an overview of principles and concepts of marrow transplantation for those who are not necessarily confronting these issues on a daily basis.

We thank all those who have given generously of their time and effort to make this book possible. We thank especially Dr. V. Gebhardt and the staff of Springer-Verlag for their responsiveness and support, Drs. T. Nevill and J. Wingard for reading the manuscript and for their suggestions, and Ms. L. Williams, B. Larson, and D. Gayle for their help with manuscript preparation and editing. We also wish to acknowledge the continued support of our teachers, especially Rainer Storb and E. Donnall Thomas.

Seattle and Vancouver
H. Joachim Deeg
Hans-Georg Klingemann
Gordon L. Phillips

Preface to the First Edition

In the late 1940s investigators observed that mice given supralethal doses of total body irradiation were protected by infusion of viable spleen or marrow cells following irradiation, and that this was accomplished by hemopoietic reconstitution with donor cells as proven using genetic markers. If a similar approach could be applied to humans, it should be possible to treat leukemia patients with any dose of chemoradiotherapy as far as nonmarrow toxicity permitted, and then rescue them by marrow transplantation. Early clinical attempts were generally unsuccessful, mostly due to a lack of knowledge of histocompatibility antigens and appropriate supportive care. These areas developed rather quickly during the 1960s, and for almost two decades now clinical marrow transplantation has been carried out with increasing success. After initially using only bone marrow from HLA indentical siblings, the field has expanded rapidly to incorporate HLA nonidentical related donors, and recently even marrow from unrelated volunteer donors. Furthermore, since for numerous patients who otherwise could benefit from transplantation a donor cannot be identified, there has been a growing interest in using the patient's own (autologous) bone marrow.

Our understanding of the principles of transplantation and our knowledge of the potential risks and benefits have quickly grown. At times it is difficult, however, to decide what is the best option for a given patient. This problem is further accentuated by the fact that the nontransplant management of the patients under consideration (e.g., patients with severe aplastic anemia, acute or chronic leukemia, lymphomas) has improved concurrently. Rather than being used in a complementary fashion, they have often been presented as competing options. Therefore, we felt that there was a need for a text that would address these issues. Conceivably, if all treatment options including bone marrow transplantation are included in treatment planning early after a patient's diagnosis is established, they can be applied more intelligently, hopefully with reduced toxicity, and hence at less risk for the patient. Consequently long-term results should improve. From a psychological point of view this may also allow a patient more time to weigh the various options and adjust to potential problems.

Although this book is directed primarily at internists and pediatricians, in particular hematologists and oncologists treating patients who might benefit bone marrow transplantation, we believe that it will also be of interest to other physicians, students and physicians in training, nurses, technologists involved in marrow transplantations, patients, and possibly those involved in insurance questions and other administrative aspects.

Our aim was to present each chapter and section in this book as a closed entity. Of necessity this has led to some overlap and duplication of sections of the discussion which appear to be pertinent in more than one place. We believe this may actually be an advantage since the readers will find any topic of interest under one heading rather than having to go through the entire book.

We are indebted to our teachers who introduced us to the exciting field of bone marrow transplantation, to our patients who gave us the gratifying experience of success, and to our colleagues and students who continue to challenge our views. We would like to thank our secretaries for their never-fatiguing support during the preparation of the manuscript, and the staff of Springer-Verlag, especially Dr. J. Wieczorek, for their responsiveness to our requests and the ability to accommodate last-minute modifications. We hope that we have not neglected any of our other duties during the preparation of the manuscript, but if we have done so we hope that the benefits of this book will allow us to make good for it.

H. JOACHIM DEEG
HANS-GEORG KLINGEMANN
GORDON L. PHILLIPS

Contents

Introduction
H.J. Deeg 1

I. Pretransplant Considerations
1. Treatment Planning and Timing of Transplantation
   H.J. Deeg and H.-G. Klingemann 7
2. Donor Selection
   H.J. Deeg 31
3. Preparation for Marrow Transplantation
   G.L. Phillips 43
4. Cost and Availability of Marrow Transplantation
   H.J. Deeg 61

II. Transplant Procedure
1. Conditioning Regimens
   G.L. Phillips 67
2. Collection, Processing and Infusion of Marrow
   H.-G. Klingemann 89

III. Acute Transplant Related Problems
1. Side Effects of Conditioning Regimens
   G.L. Phillips 105
2. Acute Graft-Versus-Host Disease (GVHD)
   H.J. Deeg 121
3. Marrow Graft Failure
   H.J. Deeg 141
4. Management of Infections
   G.L. Phillips 155

5. Interstitial Pneumonitis
      H.J. Deeg 175
   6. Hepatic Dysfunction
      H.-G. Klingemann 187
   7. Kidneys and Urinary Tract
      H.-G. Klingemann 205
   8. Central Nervous System
      H.-G. Klingemann 213

IV. **Delayed Transplant Related Problems**
   1. Follow-Up after Discharge
      from the Transplant Center
      H.J. Deeg 229
   2. Chronic Graft-Versus-Host Disease
      H.-G. Klingemann 237
   3. Pulmonary Problems
      H.-G. Klingemann 257
   4. Neuroendocrine Function, Growth,
      and Development
      H.J. Deeg 263
   5. Ophthalmologic Problems
      H.J. Deeg 269
   6. Secondary Malignancies
      H.J. Deeg 273
   7. Other Delayed Complications
      H.J. Deeg 279
   8. Rehabilitation
      H.J. Deeg 283

Outlook
H.J. Deeg 287

Glossary 295

Subject Index 299

Introduction

The goal of any anti-cancer therapy is to eradicate malignant cells and prevent their regrowth. The extent of cell kill is dependent upon the sensitivity of the cells and the dose of cytotoxic therapy administered. For many treatment modalities the dose limiting factor is myelosuppression. Hence, it is often impossible to give the maximum desired dose since patients would succumb to bone marrow aplasia and associated complications such as hemorrhage and infection. This problem can be ameliorated by the infusion of marrow following cytotoxic therapy.

Bone marrow was used for the treatment of various forms of anemia or leukemia as early as 1891. A true transplant attempt, for severe aplastic anemia, was first reported in 1939. These experiments preceded, of course, the recognition of histocompatibility antigens in man and were carried out without immunosuppressive or cytotoxic treatment of the patient. In retrospect it is, therefore, not surprising that these attempts were unsuccessful.

The observations on the effects of irradiation in atomic bomb victims in Hiroshima and Nagasaki in August 1945 resulted in a great interest in total body exposure to irradiation, and in the late 1940s several investigators began to experiment with total body irradiation (TBI) in animal models. Three dose-dependent irradiation syndromes were distinguished: the marrow syndrome (marrow aplasia with infection and hemorrhage) at doses of 500 to 700 cGy, the intestinal syndrome (bowel damage with fluid and electrolyte loss) at 1200 to 10,000 cGy, and a central nervous system (CNS) syndrome (CNS damage with seizures and uncontrolled sympathetic and parasympathetic functions) at doses >10,000 cGy. These workers also noted that mice irradiated with doses higher than those leading to marrow aplasia, but lower than those resulting in a lethal intestinal syndrome would survive if the spleen was shielded, or alternatively, if the spleen or spleen cells were transplanted to the irradiated mouse after TBI. Subsequently it was proven that hemopoietic and lymphopoietic recovery in these animals was not due to endogenous recovery of autologous cells, but rather due to the engraftment of transplanted stem cells. Similar results were achieved by using modalities other than TBI, such as cytotoxic drugs, to prepare the recipient for engraftment. Recipients carrying a lymphohemopoietic system derived from a different donor individual were called "chimeras."

It was in these animal models that most of the problems subsequently encountered in clinical transplantation were first recognized. Aside from toxicity related to the conditioning regimen, problems included hemorrhage, infection, fluid and electrolyte imbalance, and, most importantly, "secondary disease," subsequently called graft-versus-host disease (GVHD). GVHD is a syndrome observed in marrow transplant recipients given marrow from donors other than genotypically identical, monozygotic (syngeneic) twins. This reaction is initiated by donor T lymphocytes which recognize, in the recipient, histocompatibility antigens (major or minor) that differ from those present in the donor. This recognition leads to a destructive process originally directed at lymphohemopoietic cells of the recipient. Associated with this reaction are clinical manifestations in the host (patient), classically described in skin, liver, and intestinal tract, but also recognized in other tissues, for example, the conjunctivae. GVHD can be associated with substantial morbidity and mortality, due either directly to GVHD or to associated complications, especially infections. GVHD also retards the already slow postgrafting immune recovery seen in marrow transplant recipients. Consequently, efforts have been directed at preventing GVHD either by treating transplant patients with immunosuppressive agents such as methotrexate, cyclophosphamide, and cyclosporine after transplantation or by removing donor T lymphocytes from the marrow before infusion into the recipient. These approaches have improved overall transplant results, but have not been uniformly successful. In fact, the elimination of T lymphocytes from donor marrow in vitro has resulted in new problems, i.e., failure to achieve sustained engraftment even in HLA-identical transplant recipients, and increased likelihood of relapse of the underlying disease after transplantation.

The present text is meant to serve as a general guide to bone marrow transplantation. It includes considerations at the time of diagnosis, describes the process of donor selection, the actual transplant procedure, acute and chronic transplant-related problems, and long-term observations. The intent of this book is not to teach physicians how to carry out marrow transplants. Rather, this text should provide a general concept of marrow transplantation and help physicians to decide who among their patients might benefit from transplantation, when transplantation should be carried out, so as to incorporate this modality into treatment planning, and what studies should be obtained to provide a basis for discussion with and referral to a marrow transplant center. It should also help physicians in the management of potential problems that might develop posttransplant after the patient returns home. Similarly, the general nature of the text should provide background information for medical students, nurses, physician's assistants, and support staff.

Several questions such as histocompatibility typing, timing of transplantation, and toxicity in individual organs are discussed in more than one chapter. Although this has resulted in some unavoidable overlap, it also allows the readers to find relevant information in the context of various questions in which they may be interested.

References

Bortin MM, Rimm AA (1989) Increasing utilization of bone marrow transplantation. Transplantation 48:453–458
Burakoff SJ, Deeg HJ, Ferrara J, Atkinson K (eds) (1990) Graft-vs-host disease: Immunology, pathophysiology, and treatment. New York: Marcel Dekker, Inc. 1–725
O'Reilly RJ (1991) Marrow transplantation as a model system for correction of genetic disease. In: Lindsten J, Pettersson U, (eds), Etiology of Human Disease at the DNA Level, London: Raven Press, Ltd. 261–289

Philip T, Armitage JO, Spitzer G, Chauvin F, Jagannath S, Cahn J-Y, Colombat P, Goldstone AH, Gorin NC, Flesh M, Laporte J-P, Maraninchi D, Pico J, Bosly A, Anderson C, Shots R, Biron P, Cabanillas F, Dicke K (1987) High-dose therapy and autologous bone marrow transplantation after failure of conventional chemotherapy in adults with intermediate-grade or high-grade non-Hodgkin's lymphoma. N Engl J Med 316:1493

Santos GW (1983) History of bone marrow transplantation. Clin Haematol 12:611–639

Storb R. Bone marrow transplantation. In: Roitt IM, Delves PJ, (eds), Encyclopedia of Immunology, London: W.B. Saunders, Co. (in press)

Thomas ED (1990) Bone marrow transplantation – past, present and future. In: The Nobel Prizes, Stockholm: The Nobel Foundation

Thomas ED, Storb R, Clift RA, Fefer A, Johnson RL, Neiman PE, Lerner KG, Glucksberg H, Buckner CD (1975) Bone-marrow transplantation. N Engl J Med 292:832–843; 895–902

van Bekkum DW, De Vries MJ (1967) Radiation Chimeras, London: Logos Press Ltd.

I. Pretransplant Considerations

1. Treatment Planning and Timing of Transplantation

Marrow transplantation is an established modality and may represent the treatment of choice for a given patient. Hence, consideration of transplantation should be part of treatment planning early in the patient's course. However, there must be no misunderstanding: although some 30,000 patients have been transplanted, marrow transplantation remains a complex and expensive therapy. Results depend upon factors such as pretransplant therapy, disease stage, patient age, histocompatibility of donor and patient, donor and patient sex, allosensitization of the donor, donor age, and the patient's overall medical condition.

Table 1 lists diagnoses for which marrow transplantation has been carried out. Indications are constantly expanding and this list is likely to be incomplete or may include indications that are considered controversial. Nevertheless, this listing should be helpful in determining which patients may be transplant candidates.

The diagnosis of illness often generates a feeling of helplessness, and in the case of malignancy or a nonmalignant but potentially fatal disorder, evokes the impression of being doomed. There is despair, anger, and revolt against accepting such a sentence. A detailed discussion of options and prognosis is frequently helpful. Such a discussion is best led by someone experienced in the field. In fact, patients will often inquire about whom they should talk to, whom they should call, or where they could go to receive the best counseling and treatment. If a patient is already being treated at an established transplant center, these questions may not pose a problem. However, a different approach may be necessary if the patient is undergoing treatment at a medical center where transplantation is not carried out. Thus, a good coordinating effort

Table 1. Diseases treated with marrow transplantation

Acquired		Congenital
Malignant	Nonmalignant	
Acute myeloblastic leukemia	Aplastic Anemia	Immunodeficiencies
Acute lymphoblastic leukemia	Paroxysmal nocturnal hemoglobinuria	Hematologic defects
Chronic myelogenous leukemia	Myelofibrosis	Mucopolysaccharidoses
Non-Hodgkin lymphoma	Pure red cell aplasia	Mucolipidoses
Hodgkin disease	Acquired immunodeficiency syndrome	Other lysosomal diseases
Multiple myeloma		
Myelodysplastic syndrome		
Hairy cell leukemia		
Secondary leukemia		
Chronic lymphocytic leukemia		
Neuroblastoma		
Carcinoma of the breast		
Other solid tumors		

between patient, physician, and transplant center is desirable.

As soon as a patient has been identified who might benefit from marrow transplantation, the transplant option should be incorporated into the overall therapeutic plan. The age of the patient and the timing of transplantation are important considerations. Both transplant and non-transplant approaches and respective treatment results change over time. For example, as chemotherapy-induced remission and long-term disease-free survival in children with acute lymphoblastic leukemia (ALL) have improved over the years, the indication for marrow transplantation in children with ALL has been questioned. It is necessary to reevaluate and reassess the available therapeutic modalities continuously. Both transplant and non-transplant results may improve. However, if a patient relapses and presents for marrow transplantation after receiving such an aggressive chemotherapy regimen, a transplant may have less to "offer" than expected after less intensive prior chemotherapy.

Toxicity associated with marrow transplantation can be severe. The addition of new agents either to non-transplant regimens or to the transplant regimen might add further toxicity and affect transplant-related complications and quality of long-term survival. Numerous such interactions between different agents, not observed previously, have recently been reported. Similarly, various risk factors have been recognized in patients with acquired or congenital nonmalignant diseases, which will affect the timing of transplantation.

Toxicity associated with transplantation appears to increase with age. Many transplant centers restrict allogeneic transplants to patients less than 45 years of age; some have increased the age to 55 and for certain diagnoses even 65 years. While one might want to be more conservative with allogeneic transplants, it is accepted by most investigators that autologous transplants are associated with less toxicity, mainly due to the absence of GVHD, and can be carried out successfully in older patients. If autologous transplantation is not an option, non-transplant modalities might be considered in those patients.

Non-Malignant Disorders

Congenital Diseases

One of the classic indications for marrow transplantation is severe combined immunodeficiency (SCID). Children with this disease rarely live longer than one year, and marrow transplantation must be carried out early. HLA typing of the affected child, siblings, and parents should be obtained expeditiously to determine if an HLA-identical donor is available within the family. However, even if this is not the case, plans for transplantation should be pursued further. T-cell depletion of the donor marrow (see below) has allowed for successful transplantation from a haploidentical parent. Furthermore, if for some reason the parents cannot serve as marrow donors, it may be possible to identify an unrelated volunteer donor who is HLA phenotypically matched with the patient. In a small number of children, fetal liver cell transplantation has been attempted, and engraftment of T cells (but often not of B cells) has been reported.

There are additional congenital immunodeficiencies which can be approached similarly. These include SCID with ADA deficiency, the bare lymphocyte syndrome, iodophor responsive combined immunodeficiency, combined immunodeficiency with capping abnormality, nucleoside phosphorylase deficiency, leukocyte adhesion defects and others. In patients with ADA deficiency it has been difficult to achieve consistent engraftment. Generally, the presence of strong natural killer cell activity before transplantation was correlated with graft failure.

Most important in all these patients is the prevention of infection prior to transplantation, since the presence of infection will substantially increase mortality after transplantation. As soon as a diagnosis of immunodeficiency is established, or only suspected, an experienced transplant center should be contacted for further management of the patient.

There are other congenital immunodeficiency disorders which usually are compatible with a somewhat longer survival. These include the Wiskott-Aldrich syndrome, chronic granulomatous disease, ataxia-telangiectasia, cartilage-hair hypoplasia, and others listed in Table 2. These diagnoses may allow for more time to observe the patient, and evaluate siblings (if available) and parents before a decision for transplantation is made. In contrast to patients with combined immunodeficiencies, these patients generally require immunosuppressive conditioning (by drugs or irradiation or a combination of both) to achieve sustained engraftment even with HLA-identical bone marrow. Hence, pretransplant treatment in any form, including blood product transfusions, may well have an effect on the toxicity and efficacy associated with conditioning for marrow transplantation.

Metabolic storage diseases have also been treated successfully by marrow transplantation. Some of these disorders are listed in Table 2. Only very few patients with any one of these diseases have been transplanted; generally they have achieved sustained engraftment. GVHD has developed in several patients. While excellent enzyme correction and clinical improvement have been observed with some disorders

Table 2. Congenital disorders treated by marrow transplantation

Immunodeficiencies – Severe combined immunodeficiency (SCID) – Combined immunodeficiency (CID) 　– Reticular dysgenesis 　– Cartilage-hair hypoplasia 　– Bare lymphocyte syndrome – Leukocyte adhesion defects (LAD) – Actin deficiency – Chronic mucocutaneous candidiasis – Others Hematologic defects – Wiscott-Aldrich Syndrome – Fanconi Anemia – Blackfan-Diamond Anemia – Thalassemia – Sickle cell disease – Glanzman thrombasthenia – Congenital amegakaryocytosis – Thrombocytopenia-absent radius (TAR) syndrome – Familial erythrophagocytic lymphohistocytosis (FEL) – Gaucher disease – Chronic granulomatous disease – Congenital neutropenia – Chediak Higashi Syndrome Osteopetrosis	Mucopolysaccaridoses – Hurler Syndrome – Hunter Syndrome – Maroteaux-Lamy Syndrome – Others Mucolipidoses – Metachromatic leukodystrophy – Other lipidoses – Adrenokeukodystrophy Other lysosomal diseases – Lesch-Nyhan Syndrome – Type IIa glycogen storage disease

(e.g., Hurler disease, Gaucher disease), other defects (e.g., Lesch-Nyhan syndrome, GMI gangliosidosis) cannot be easily corrected.

In patients with Fanconi anemia, transplants have generally been carried out when severe marrow aplasia and pancytopenia developed. Toxicity associated with transplantation (e.g., mucositis, cystitis) has often been more severe than in patients with related diagnoses (e.g., idiopathic severe aplastic anemia). In an attempt to reduce toxicity, conditioning regimens have been modified, for example, by moderately reducing the dose of cyclophosphamide or by drastically reducing cyclophosphamide (from 200 mg/kg to 20 mg/kg) and adding thoracoabdominal irradiation (see conditioning regimens below). Failure of engraftment has not been a problem in patients transplanted from an HLA-identical sibling but has been observed with T-cell depleted marrow, especially from an HLA-incompatible related or unrelated donor.

An alternative approach has recently been reported: Following genetic counseling, parents of patients with Fanconi anemia decided to have another baby who might serve as donor for the affected child. This fetus, HLA type and chromosome fragility were determined and, if appropriate, umbilical cord blood was obtained at the time of delivery and used for transplantation. It is too early to assess what the success with this approach will be. Also, numerous ethical concerns have been raised and need to be addressed.

One should consider that patients with Fanconi anemia are at a significant risk of developing secondary malignancies including leukemia even if they do not develop marrow hypoplasia. These diseases have also been treated by marrow transplantation, albeit less successfully, and it might be preferable to treat the patient earlier, at a time when there is no evidence of clonal evolution and malignant transformation.

Although genetic counseling has substantially reduced the frequency of births of babies with homozygous thalassemia, still many such children are born. Pending progress at the level of molecular manipulation, bone marrow transplantation offers the only curative therapy. It is important to consult, early in the patient's course, a transplant physician who has experience with this disease. Lucarelli and colleagues have recently shown that patients with thalassemia major who have received adequate chelation therapy and do not have hepatomegaly and portal fibrosis fare significantly better after transplantation than patients with these three risk factors (survival after transplantation from an HLA-identical sibling, 95% versus 55%, respectively). These data suggest, therefore, that transplantation should be carried out early in the disease course. It also seems prudent to recommend judicious transfusion support and to avoid sensitization. These considerations are important since both the nature of the disease, with a "turned-on" hypercellular marrow, and the sensitization status of the patient may interfere with marrow engraftment. Although this is not a malignant disease, the abnormal hemopoietic stem cells apparently have a growth advantage. They are at times difficult to eradicate, and thalassemia can recur after transplantation.

Several children with sickle-cell disease have been transplanted successfully; however, it is currently controversial what the criteria for transplantation in these patients should be.

Severe Aplastic Anemia

Aplastic anemia is a nonmalignant but often lethal disease of heterogeneous etiology. At the present time basically two modalities of treatment are available:

a) immunosuppression, usually in the form of antithymocyte globulin (ATG), cyclosporine, glucocorticoid, or combinations of those agents; and
b) marrow transplantation.

Some centers have reported very encouraging results with immunosuppression, with response rates of 40–60% and a probability of survival of 50–70%. Hemopoiesis, when tested in vitro, remains abnormal, and late recurrences of marrow aplasia and the development of myelodysplasia, acute leukemia or paroxysmal nocturnal hemoglobinuria have been observed. The use of hemopoietic growth factors (see below) has met with only limited success and usually in patients who still had preserved low levels of hemopoiesis.

In general, survival is superior with marrow transplantation. Due to the nature of the disease, autologous transplantation is not an option; a healthy allogeneic (or in rare instances, syngeneic) donor must be available. In earlier studies patients with aplastic anemia were found to have a very high probability of marrow graft rejection, ranging from 30–60% even after transplantation from an HLA identical sibling. Most analyses indicate that rejection was usually due to transfusion-induced sensitization of the patient before marrow transplant; subsequent studies showed that untransfused patients were, indeed, significantly less likely to reject the marrow graft and approximately 90% of these patients are surviving with sustained engraftment. Hence, it is desirable to carry out transplants in untransfused patients. This implies that any physician diagnosing a patients with severe aplastic anemia should, whenever possible, avoid transfusions and expeditiously obtain HLA typing on the patient, siblings, and other family members so that the patient can be referred to a transplant center for transplantation while still untransfused. If the patient must be transfused, family members should not be used as donors and leukocyte-poor preparations should be given. In every-day practice most patients with severe aplastic anemia will have been transfused when they present for transplantation. Because of the historically very high incidence of graft rejection with conventional conditioning regimens, more aggressive regimens have been developed (II.1), and if an HLA identical donor can be identified within the family a transplant should be carried out at least in patients 45 years of age or younger. With currently used conditioning regimens (see II.1) approximately 90–95% of patients achieve sustained engraftment, and 80%–90% of patients can be expected to become longterm survivors.

If patients do not have an HLA identical related donor or are older than 45 years, the situation is different. In older patients allogeneic transplants are associated with more toxicity than in younger patients, and after HLA non-identical transplants the incidences of both graft failure and GVHD are high. As a result longterm survival in both patient groups is inferior to that seen with HLA identical transplants in younger patients. Therefore, first line therapy for these patients generally should be immunosuppressive therapy. Only if they fail to respond, generally within 2–3 months of initiation of such therapy, should they be considered for marrow transplantation. Because of the prolonged interval of pancytopenia in these patients infections and hemorrhagic complications are more likely and results are expected to be inferior.

However, the lack of an HLA-identical sibling per se is not reason enough to abandon the possibility of marrow transplantation. Several transplants from HLA phenotypically identical unrelated volunteer donors have been reported, and a search should be initiated, particularly if the patient's HLA

Table 3. Common HLA – A, B halotypes and B/DR associations[a]

HLA-A, B	B, DR Linkage[b]
Caucasians:	
A1, B8	B8, DR3
A3, B7	B7, DR2
A2, Bw62	B62, DR4
A2, Bw60	Bw60, DR4
A3, Bw35	Bw35, DR1 (DR5)
A29, Bw44	Bw44, DR7 (DR4)
A1, Bw57	Bw57, DR7
A25, B18	B18, DR5 (DR3)
Negroids:	
A1, B8	B8, DR3
A30, Bw42	Bw42, DR3
A28, Bw64	Bw64, DR7
A2, Bw58	Bw58, DR11
A28, Bw58	Bw58, DR14
A3, B7	B7, DR2
A2, B7	B7, DR2
Japanese:	
Aw24, Bw52	Bw52, DR2
Aw24, B7	B7, DR1
Aw33, Bw44	Bw44, DRw14
Aw24, Bw54	Bw54, DR4
A2, Bw46	Bw46, DRw8
Aw24, Bw35	Bw35, DR4 (DRw8)

[a] listed in order of decreasing frequency.
[b] most frequent (second most frequent) associated DR allele.

haplotypes are common in a given population (Table 3). Further, several transplants have been carried out, usually from related donors, who were not completely HLA-identical, but differed for at least one HLA antigen. This usually required more severe immunosuppression of the patient, generally in the form of TBI, but successful engraftment and long-term survival have been achieved.

What has been said for severe aplastic anemia in general also applies to paroxysmal nocturnal hemoglobinuria, once the patient develops failure of one or more cell lines.

Malignant Diseases

Myelodyplastic Syndrome (MDS)

Patients with MDS who have an HLA identical or one antigen mismatched related donor and are 55 years of age or younger should be transplanted without delay. In older patients, one may want to provide supportive therapy to those with the diagnostic subcategories refractory anemia (RA) without or with ring sideroblasts (RARS) and transplant only those with refractory anemia with excess blasts (RAEB) and those in transformation (RAEBT) or with chronic myelomonocytic leukemia (CMML). Particularly patients with RA or RARS must be distinguished from patients with classic severe aplastic anemia since a more aggressive (anti-leukemic) regimen is required to eradicate the disease. This can usually be achieved by morphologic and cytogenetic analysis and if necessary by applying molecular biology tools to determine whether clonal hemopoiesis, suggesting a malignant disorder is present. Patients whose marrow shows severe fibrosis may be at risk of graft failure (see III.3).

If no family donor can be identified an unrelated donor search should be undertaken; next to CML, MDS is currently the most widely accepted diagnosis for transplantation from an unrelated donor.

Recently attempts at transplantation of autologous peripheral blood stem cells have been made; however, this must be considered highly experimental.

Acute Myeloblastic Leukemia (AML)

Very aggressive and effective combination chemotherapy, usually involving the use of cytosine arabinoside and daunorubicin or related drugs, has resulted in complete remission in 70–80% of pediatric and adult patients; it has been claimed that with chemotherapy alone, as many as 50% of patients, especially among children or in adults with subtypes of AML such as FAB M3 or chromosome 16 abnormalities and eosinophilia, may be cured. Thus, it may be difficult to select patients who should be transplanted. On the other hand, most studies in adults suggest that about 25% of patients achieve a prolonged unmaintained remission after chemotherapy alone.

In the early days of marrow transplantation, all transplants were carried out in patients with far advanced, usually chemotherapy-resistant disease. Encouraged by results in these endstage patients, several transplant teams began in the mid-1970s to transplant patients earlier in their course, preferentially in chemotherapy-induced first remission (see I.2.). This approach has resulted in long-term disease-free survival of approximately 50–60% in adults and 60–70% in children. Nevertheless, 10–20% of transplanted patients still succumb to recurrent leukemia.

What is the best approach at the present time? At the time of diagnosis or as soon as chemotherapy-induced remission is achieved, HLA typing of parents, siblings, and possibly children, should be obtained. A transplant center should be contacted. If an HLA-identical sibling or a family member differing from the patient by only one HLA antigen is available, and the patient is not more than 55 years of age, the patient should be referred for allogeneic marrow transplantation. However, as indicated above, selected groups of patients have a reasonably good prognosis with conventional chemotherapy. In addition, recent retrospective analyses suggest that the relapse rate of patients transplanted for AML in early relapse may not be significantly higher than the relapse rate observed after transplantation in first remission. If this is the case, one might argue that one should induce patients into remission and observe without transplant. If relapse occurs, transplantation should be carried out as expeditiously as possible. Relapse-free survival with transplantation at this point has been approximately 25%, and in recent studies with only short follow-up, about 40%. The combined probabilities of relapse-free survival with chemotherapy alone plus survival with transplantation after first relapse might then be around 60%, i.e., comparable to that observed with transplantation in first remission. This approach is particularly attractive in older patients who generally experience substantial transplant-related toxicity. However, so far no controlled study has been reported, and at the present time transplantation while in first remission still appears to offer the best results at least in patients up to about 40 years of age.

If a patient fails to achieve a first remission or relapses, marrow transplantation offers a better outlook than chemotherapy, although the probability of disease-free survival is at best 20%. It should be pointed out that many established transplant centers are reluctant to accept patients in relapse, or assign a low priority on their waiting lists, which may not be in the patient's best interest. Results obtained with related donors mismatched for more than one HLA antigen are generally poor, and an autologous transplant or an allogeneic transplant from a matched unrelated donor could be considered, especially in those patients who have a disease at high risk of relapse (e.g., FAB type M5, certain cytogenetic abnormalities or high white blood cell count at diagnosis). Unfortunately, the search time to find an unrelated donor may be 3 to 6 months and many patients will relapse before a donor can be identified. Autologous BMT offers an alternative for those patients. Hence if a preliminary search does not identify potential unrelated donor, an autologous marrow should be harvested and an autologous transplant should be performed either in first remission or at the time of relapse. However, if potential donors are identified in the registry, final typing results should be awaited and, if necessary, the patient should be given additional consolidation chemotherapy. In patients with "standard-risk" AML, most centers offer conventional chemotherapy and consider autologous or matched unrelated donor transplantation only at the time of relapse or in second or subsequent remission.

Contrary to some of the congenital disorders, or acquired severe aplastic anemia, transfusion prior to transplantation does not appear to be a major risk factor for the outcome after marrow transplantation.

Acute Lymphoblastic Leukemia (ALL)

Several chemotherapeutic regimens developed in Europe and the United States have achieved complete remissions in more than 90% of pediatric and about 70% for adult patients with ALL. However, the prognosis varies dependent upon patient age, presentation of the disease, immunophenotype, cytogenetic abnormalities and other factors.

Adult patients with newly diagnosed ALL may belong to high or standard-risk groups. Assignment to the high-risk groups is based on the following criteria:

- White blood cell count >50 and 10^9/L at diagnosis
- Presence of the Philadelphia chromosome
- B or null cell immunophenotype
- Prolonged time to achieve first complete remission
- Age of patient >20 years
- Presence of a mediastinal mass at diagnosis
- CNS involvement at presentation

Adult patients who belong to a high-risk group should receive an allogeneic transplant in first remission if a suitable donor is available. Some small series suggest a probability of relapse-free survival of approximately 50%. If patients are transplanted in a subsequent remission or while in relapse the probability of longterm disease free survival decreases to 20–30%.

If a related allogeneic donor is not available, storage and transplantation of autologous marrow or transplantation from an HLA matched unrelated donor can be considered. There is currently no agreement as to which approach is preferable or superior.

Autologous marrow is generally subjected to in vitro purging with appropriate monoclonal antibodies, chemical agents or both. Leukemia-free survival has been reported at 10–50%, dependent upon disease stage, time of marrow harvest and phenotype. As more refined studies on minimal residual disease are being carried out, it is likely that results with truly leukemia-free marrow will improve. Results will then depend upon completeness of eradication of leukemia in the patient and should be comparable to those obtained with allogeneic marrow, except, of course, for the fact that the antileukemic effect of allogeneic cells is lacking.

Results with the use of marrow from unrelated donors are limited; currently, they appear to be comparable to those obtained with autologous marrow, although the causes of failure differ (GVHD versus recurrence of leukemia).

The situation in children is slightly different insofar as current treatment protocols produce longterm survival even in a high proportion of children with less favorable prognosis. However, allogeneic transplantation is appropriate for children who relapse while receiving appropriate maintenance chemotherapy or in children with testicular or CNS relapse. Furthermore, FAB L3 morphology (Burkitt type) or the presence of a Philadelphia chromosome or a 4:11 translocation carry a poor prognosis with conventional chemotherapy and should be transplanted while in first remission. Children with standard-risk disease are often transplanted in second remissions. This strategy might be challenged, however, by some investigators who have achieved excellent chemotherapy results with disease-free survival in excess of 50% in children who were induced into a second remission. What has been said about autologous and unrelated transplants in adults generally also applies to children.

When treating a patient with ALL, and considering the possibility of subsequent marrow transplantation, one should attempt to avoid CNS toxicity induced by the initial treatment. In particular, pediatric patients who are given cerebrospinal or cranial irradiation (usually 1800 to 2400 cGy) have an increased risk of developing leukoencephalopathy after transplantation. Toxicity is further increased by the concurrent intrathecal administration of methotrexate. Thus, if a patient is a candidate for early transplantation, conceivably cranial irradiation should be avoided and CNS treatment and prophylaxis should be limited to chemotherapy (methotrexate, cytosine arabinoside, dexamethasone) only. This may be important not only in regard to leukoencephalopathy, but also in regard to longitudinal growth and overall development in children. Cranial irradiation, especially if followed later by total body irradiation, clearly impairs growth, and intellectual and emotional development.

Chronic Myelogenous Leukemia (CML)

A donor search should always be initiated in patients up to 55 and possibly 65 years of age diagnosed with CML. Currently, no modality other than marrow transplantation offers the possibility of cure for CML. Treatment with recombinant human interferon results in cytogenetic remission in 25–30% of patients. In some patients, this remission may last for years; however, it is presently not clear whether survival for the entire group will be prolonged. Of course, physicians and patients will want to exploit the option of interferon treatment. It should be pointed out, however, that several groups observed the best transplant results in patients transplanted within one year of diagnosis. With transplantation from an HLA identical or one antigen mismatched related donor within one year of diagnosis survival rates of 70–90% have been reported. Patients in chronic phase transplanted with marrow from an HLA matched unrelated donor currently have a 40% probability of longterm survival.

If transplantation is delayed the probability of cure decreases, and with transplants in accelerated phase or blast transformation only 25% and 15% of patients respectively have become longterm survivors. Recent data suggest that as many as 40% of patients in accelerated phase may survive longterm if prepared with an aggressive conditioning regimen. Since outcome with HLA nonidentical transplantation is generally poorer, patients who do not have an HLA identical donor are often transplanted in a more advanced stage of their disease. If patients who have undergone blast transformation achieve a second chronic phase following chemotherapy, their chances of becoming longterm survivors after transplantation may be 40%.

Autologous transplantation in patients with CML has been attempted by several investigators. Generally marrow was harvested and cryopreserved during chronic phase. Once the patient's disease accelerated, the patient was conditioned for transplant and the chronic phase marrow was infused. As a rule, the post-transplant chronic phase was short and correlated with the time elapsed between marrow harvest and disease acceleration. More recently investigators have harvested marrow from CML patients and cultured in vitro. Under certain conditions cells of the malignant clone die in culture. Conceivably marrow so treated can be used for autologous transplantation if normal stem cells are left intact. This approach is experimental, and some variations are currently being explored.

It appears that prolonged pretransplant treatment with busulfan represents a risk factor for outcome after marrow transplantation. Hence, a patient who has been identified as a transplant candidate should preferentially be treated with hydroxyurea to avoid the impact of busulfan on post transplant complications. Some studies suggest that splenomegaly is a negative prognostic factor, and that pre-transplant splenectomy might improve the outlook in regard to both survival and GVHD; however, this issue remains controversial.

Non-Hodgkin Lymphoma

Effective curative therapy other than transplantation is available for most patients with Hodgkin disease and for some types of non-Hodgkin lymphoma. However, the probability of cure is low, e.g., in patients with non-Hodgkin lymphoma of aggressive (high grade) histology, either a priori or once they have relapsed from first remission. These patients should be considered for marrow transplantation, either with autologous marrow (if the marrow is not involved or can be purged) or from an HLA-identical or one-antigen different allogeneic donor. It is currently unclear which approach is superior. Prior irradiation, particularly to the mediastinum, represents a significant risk factor for the postgrafting development of interstitial pneumonitis.

In patients with non-Hodgkin lymphoma, involvement of the CNS, the marrow or both at the time of diagnosis are associated with early relapse and poor survival. Lymphoblastic lymphomas of the convoluted cell type also have a very poor prognosis with conventional chemotherapy alone. Nodular poorly differentiated lymphocytic lymphoma, although relatively indolent in its course, is unlikely to be cured by chemotherapy. In these patients allogeneic marrow transplantation from a suitable related donor might be carried out early in the disease course and even in first remission. Alternatively, if the marrow is cleared or can be purged by appropriate agents, autologous marrow can be cryopreserved and used at the time of relapse or immediately, analogous to allogeneic marrow. Dependent upon histology and disease stage, 25%–85% of patients may be cured of their disease. In patients in so-called "sensitive relapse" (i.e., disease responsive to chemotherapy), disease-free survival of approximately 40% can be achieved. Conversely, patients who have a "resistant relapse" are unlikely to benefit and should not be considered for marrow transplantation. Patients who do not achieve a complete remission, relapse early after a full course of first-line chemotherapy or progress during induction chemotherapy are also candidates for marrow grafting. Among patients with large cell (cleaved or non-cleaved) lymphoma 70% of those who achieve a complete remission with chemotherapy survive disease-free beyond 5 years. Thus transplantation should be reserved to those who fail to achieve remission or relapse.

Hodgkin Disease

Patients with Hodgkin disease should be transplanted, generally with autologous marrow, if they fail induction therapy or relapse from remission achieved with optimum chemotherapy (MOPP + ABVD). Survival is 50%–70%. If initial chemotherapy was "less than optimum" and relapse occurred after a prolonged remission interval it may be appropriate to induce another remission with chemo- or radiochemotherapy.

Patients who show marrow involvement at presentation have a poor prognosis. If remission can be induced they should have their marrow cryopreserved and either be transplanted as consolidation therapy or at the first sign of relapse. If the marrow does not clear or a suitable donor is available an allogeneic transplant should be carried out. Autologous peripheral blood stem cells may offer an alternative, although this approach must currently be considered experimental.

If neither of the above approaches is acceptable, an HLA identical unrelated transplant should be considered.

Multiple Myeloma

Multiple myeloma frequently affects patients more than 50 years of age, but occurs in younger age groups as well. Conventional treatment is non-curative, and median survival is only 2–3 years. It was thought, therefore, that these patients might benefit from marrow transplantation. Both allogeneic and autologous transplants have been carried out. The optimum time for transplantation is not known. In the past, generally only patients who failed two standard chemotherapy regimens were accepted for transplantation; for autologous transplants investigators prefer marrow which contains less than 30% plasma cells. Recently there has been interest in transplanting patients with a lower tumor burden earlier in their course.

Current data suggest that 60% of patients show responses after allogeneic transplantation, and 35–40% survive in remission or without requiring maintenance chemotherapy. The mechanism by which autologous transplantation improves patient outcome is not clear; however, some autologous recipients have shown unmaintained responses extending beyond 2 years.

Solid Tumors

The place of marrow transplantation in the treatment of solid tumors is not clearly defined. Many solid tumors, such as metastic melanoma, carcinoma of the lung, carcinoma of the breast, recurrent non-seminomatous germ cell tumors are not curable with currently available chemotherapy and offer areas in which to explore the usefulness of marrow transplantation.

The major focus of ongoing studies is breast cancer. Both women with stage IV disease, usually after having received conventional chemotherapy, and women considered at high risk at the time of diagnosis (e.g., more than 10 axillary nodes involved by metastases), have been transplanted with autologous marrow. This approach is highly experimental and it would be premature to draw conclusions.

Some success has been achieved in children with extensive neuroblastoma, and in patients with non-seminomatous testicular tumors.

Other Indications

The place of marrow transplantation for the treatment of the acquired immunodeficiency syndrome (AIDS) and associated lymphoma remains to be determined. Similarly, the usefulness of marrow transplantation in victims of radiation accidents remains to be proven.

Patient Consultation

Initially, marrow transplantation was applied only at a very few centers. No trained physicians were available outside those centers, and patients had little access to information pertaining to this potentially lifesaving therapy. Since many established and conventionally trained hematologists and oncologists considered the procedure, quite appropriately, experimental, this modality became available very gradually to only small numbers of patients. Over the last decade, however, many referring physicians have taken advantage of the availability of an increasing number of centers with growing expertise in marrow transplantation, and have sent patients for consultation before a decision about marrow transplantation was reached.

This approach has some disadvantages, such as the cost of traveling and a considerable time investment on the part of both patient and physician. However, advantages far outweigh disadvantages. Consultation with a physician at a marrow transplant center allows the patient to ask, and more importantly, to obtain answers to questions that could not be well answered elsewhere. It is also possible to provide the patient with recent information not yet published, or publicized. Furthermore, results can be put into perspective better by a transplant physician than by someone not involved in this field.

Very importantly, a patient and any accompanying family member, possibly the potential marrow donor, can visit with patients who are undergoing or recovering from transplantation. This allows for more immediate insight into the psychological stress and other problems associated with transplantation and often helps the patient to prepare better for transplantation. In addition to the physician's expertise, discussions with nurses and other support personnel are helpful. Patients can meet a social worker to obtain information regarding other potential problems and discuss living arrangements, insurance coverage, and posttransplant problems. Finally, if patients are eventually transplanted, and are transplanted at that particular center, they will have already familiarized themselves with the environment, and possibly with nurses and physicians who subsequently will be taking care of them. Such an approach reduces the apprehension and fear associated with marrow transplantation in many albeit not all patients, by receiving positive feedback from patients who have gone through the procedure, have done well, and have again developed a positive outlook on life. Often this has been crucial for the determination of patients to proceed with this very involved, expensive treatment, which is still associated with a high probability of morbidity and often mortality.

Where Should a Patient Be Transplanted?

In the early and mid-1970s few bone marrow transplant units existed. Currently there are between 200 and 300 institutions worldwide where bone marrow transplantation is being performed. However, this must not be interpreted as an indication that marrow transplantation should be carried out at any hospital where a patient with a disease amenable to transplantation is being diagnosed or treated. The resources and support services required for marrow transplantation are considerable, and can be used efficiently and successfully at an individual center only if a sufficiently large number of patients is being transplanted, although it is a matter of debate what this number should be.

From a technical point of view the actual marrow transplant is a rather simple procedure, however, the ramifications, and the potential complications associated with it are complex. Problems appear to be more severe with more advanced disease, prolonged disease duration, higher patient age and histoincompatible transplants, requiring more expertise and a broader support system. The number of well trained marrow transplant physicians experienced with all aspects of this procedure is limited. As a result many smaller transplant units have carefully selected patients to be transplanted, i.e., have limited transplantation to good risk patients. Poor risk patients, who usually have no other alternative, may be referred to larger centers for consideration for transplantation. Results reported from the respective centers are, therefore, likely to differ. A physician considering referral of a patient for bone marrow transplantation should be aware of this.

However, despite considerable progress, many problems remain even at large transplant centers. Answers to the open questions can be obtained only in controlled studies conducted by experienced investigators and involving sufficiently large numbers of patients at single or multiple institutions. The more expeditiously patients are accrued to these studies, the faster answers will be obtained, leading to improved survival in future patients. At the same time it is true that many of the larger transplant centers have long waiting lists for patients which may also lead to biased selection. From a cost/benefit standpoint this is understandable. However, it is of no help to the individual patient. Therefore, a sound approach for any physician taking care of a potential marrow transplant candidate would be to call several marrow transplant centers, perhaps one nearby and (if different) one of the large centers, in order to form for himself an opinion as to what the best approach for his patient may be.

References

Appelbaum FR, Barral J, Storb R, Fisher LD, Schoch G, Ramberg RE, Shulman H, Anasetti C, Bearman I, Beatty P, Bensinger WI, Buckner D, Clift RA, Hansen JA, Martin P, Finn B, Petersen FB, Sanders JE, Singer J, Stewart P, Sullivan KM, Witherspoon RP, Thomas ED (1990) Bone marrow transplantation for patients with myelodysplasia. Pretreatment variables and outcome. Ann Int Med 112:590–597

Armitage JO. Bone marrow transplantation in the treatment of patients with lymphoma (1989) Blood 73:1749

Baranov A, Gale RP, Guskova A, Piatkin E, Selidovkin G, Muravyova L, Champlin RE, Danilova N, Yevseeva L, Petrosyan L, Pushkareva S, Konchalovsky M, Gordeeva A, Protasova T, Reisner Y, Mickey MR, Terasaki PI (1989) Bone marrow transplantation after the Chernobyl nuclear accident. N Engl J Med 321:205–212

Beatty PG, Clift RA, Mickelson EM, Nisperos BB, Flournoy N, Martin PJ, Sanders JE, Stewart P, Buckner CD, Storb R, Thomas ED, Hansen JA (1985) Marrow transplantation from related donors other than HLA-identical siblings. N Engl J Med 313:765

Berman E, Little C, Gee T, O'Reilly R, Clarkson B (1992) Reasons that patients with acute myelogenous leukemia do not undergo allogeneic bone marrow transplantation. N Engl J Med 326:156–160

Champlin RE, Horowitz MM, van Bekkum DW, et al. (1989) Graft failure following bone marrow transplantation for severe aplastic anemia: Risk factors and treatment results. Blood 73:606

Chao NJ, Forman SJ, Schmidt GM, et al. (1991) Allogeneic bone marrow transplantation for high-risk acute lymphoblastic leukemia during first complete remission. Blood 78:1923

Cheson BD, Lacerna L, Leyland-Jones B, Sarosy G, Wittes RE (1989) Autologous bone marrow transplantation. Current status and future directions. Ann Intern Med 110:51–65

Deeg HJ, Self S, Storb R, et al. (1986) Decreased incidence of marrow graft rejection in patients with severe aplastic anemia: Changing impact of risk factors. Blood 68:1363

Fischer A, Durnady A, de Villartay J-P, Vilmer E, Le Deist F, Gerota I, Griscelli C (1986) HLA-Haploidentical bone marrow transplantation for severe combined immunodeficiency using E Rosette fractionation and cyclosporine. Blood 67:444–449

Flowers MED, Doney KC, Storb R, Deeg HJ, Sanders JE, Sullivan KM, Bryant E, Witherspoon RP, Appelbaum FR, Buckner CD, Hansen JA, Thomas ED (1992) Marrow transplantation for Fanconi anemia with or without leukemic transformation: An update of the Seattle experience. Bone Marrow Transplantation 9:167–173

Gahrton G, Tura S, Ljungman P, et al. (1991) Allogeneic bone marrow transplantation in multiple myeloma. N Engl J Med 325:1267

Gluckman E, Broxmeyer HE, Auerbach AD, Friedman HS, Douglas GW, Devergie A, Esperou H, Thierry D, Socie G, Lehn P, Cooper S, English D, Kurtzberg J, Bard J, Boyse EA (1989) Hematopoietic reconstitution in a patient with Fanconi's anemia by means of umbilical-cord blood from an HLA-identical sibling. N Engl J Med 321:1174–1178

Horowitz MM, Messerer D, Hoelzer D, Gale RP, Neiss A, Atkinson K, Barrett AJ, Büchner T, Freund M, Heil G, Hiddemann W, Kolb H-J,

Löffler H, Marmont AM, Maschmeyer G, Rimm AA, Rozman C, Sobocinski KA, Speck B, Thiel E, Weisdorf DJ, Zwaan FE, Bortin MM (1991) Chemotherapy compared with bone marrow transplantation for adults with acute lymphoblastic leukemia in first remission. Ann Intern Med 115:13-18

Klingemann H-G, Storb R, Fefer A, et al. (1986) Bone marrow transplantation in patients aged 45 years and older. Blood 67:770

Krivit W, Whitley CB, Chang PN et al. (1989) Lysosomal storage diseases treated by bone marrow transplantation. Bone marrow transplantation, current controversies, RP Gale, R Champlin (eds), A R Liss Inc, New York

Lane HC, Zunich KM, Wilson W, Cefali F, Easter M, Kovacs JA, Masur H, Leitman SF, Klein HG, Steis RG, Longo DL, Fauci AS (1990) Syngeneic bone marrow transplantation and adoptive transfer of peripheral blood lymphocytes combined with zidovudine in human immunodeficiency virus (HIV) infection. Ann Intern Med 113:512-519

Linker CA, Levitt LJ, O'Donnell M, Forman SJ, Ries CA (1991) Treatment of adult acute lymphoblastic leukemia with intensive cyclical chemotherapy: A follow-up report. Blood 78:2814-2822

Lucarelli G, Galimberti M, Polchi P, Angelucci E, Baronciani D, Giardini C, Politi P, Durzaai SMT, Muretto P, Albertini F (1990) Bone marrow transplantation in patients with thalassemia. N Engl J Med 322:417-421

Moore MAS, Castro-Malaspina H (1991) Immunosuppression in aplastic anemia – postponing the inevitable? N Engl J Med 324:1358-1360

Reece DE, Barnett MJ, Connors JM, et al. (1991) Intensive chemotherapy with cyclophosphamide, carmustine, and etoposide followed by autologous bone marrow transplantation for relapsed Hodgkin's disease. J Clin Oncol 9:1871

Santos GW (1989) Marrow Transplantation in acute nonlymphocytic leukemia. Blood 74:901-908

Simon W, Segel GB, Lichtman MA (1988) Upper and lower time limits in the decision to recommend marrow transplantation for patients with chronic myelogenous leukaemia. Br J Haematol 70:31-36

Speck B, Gratwohl A, Nissen C, Osterwalder B, Wursch A, Tichelli A, Lori A, Reusser P, Jeannet M, Signer E (1986) Treatment of severe aplastic anemia. Exp Hematol 14:126

Storb R, Anasetti C, Appelbaum F, Bensinger W, Buckner CD, Clift R, Deeg HJ, Doney K, Hansen J, Loughran T, Martin P, Pepe M, Petersen F, Sanders J, Singer J, Stewart P, Sullivan KM, Witherspoon R, Thomas ED (1991) Marrow transplantation for severe aplastic anemia and thalassemia major. Semin Hematol 28:235-239

Thomas ED, Clift RA, Fefer A, Appelbaum FR, Beatty P, Bensinger WI, Buckner CD, Cheever MA, Deeg HJ, Doney K, Flournoy N, Greenberg P, Hansen JA, Martin P, McGuffin R, Ramberg R, Sanders JE, Singer J, Stewart P, Storb R, Sullivan K, Weiden PL, Witherspoon R (1986) Marrow transplantation for the treatment of chronic myelogenous leukemia. Ann Int Med 104:155

Tichelli A, Gratwohl A, Wursch A, Nissen C, Speck B (1988) Late haematological complications in severe aplastic anaemia. Br J Haematol 69:413-418

2. Donor Selection

Source of Marrow

Dependent upon the patient's disease, there may be one or several options when selecting a marrow source (Tables 4 and 5).

Family Donors

In contrast to solid organ transplants, a marrow transplant is generally from a related (family) donor, preferably identical with the patient for the major histocompatibility complex (MHC) encoded human leukocyte antigens (HLA) i.e., usually a sibling. However, the donor may also be an HLA-nonidentical family member, or in rare instances, a monozygotic (identical) twin. An identical twin is theoretically the ideal donor, combining the advantages of autologous marrow (no histocompatibility barrier) and allogeneic marrow (normal hemopoietic cells: no tumor contamination); however, as will be discussed below, there may also be certain disadvantages. From this pool of relatives, a suitable donor can be found for approximately 35% of patients. This is unsatisfactory, and efforts have been made in two directions to allow for the option of transplantation for a larger proportion of patients.

Unrelated Donors

In the late 1970s several investigators showed that some patients who did not have a suitable marrow donor within the family could be transplanted successfully with marrow obtained from an unrelated volunteer. This was possible if the unrelated individual expressed HLA alleles which were very similar or

Table 4. Potential marrow sources for different disease categories[a]

Disease: Acquired, usually malignant diseases with intact hemopoietic stem cell function
Potential Marrow Source:
    Allogeneic
    Syngeneic
    Autologous[b]
Disease: Acquired diseases affecting hemopoietic function
Potential Marrow Source:
    Allogeneic
    Syngeneic
Disease: Congenital diseases
Potential Marrow Source:
    Allogeneic[c]

---

[a] excluding the possibility of xenogeneic marrow.
[b] peripheral blood stem cells may be an alternative.
[c] umbilical cord blood has been used in some patients.

Table 5. Potential marrow donors

Autologous: Patient's own marrow
Syngeneic: Monozygotic (identical) twin
Allogeneic: HLA genotypically identical sibling
    HLA phenotypically identical donor
      – Sibling
      – Parent
      – Other family member
      – Unrelated volunteer
    HLA nonidentical donor
      – Family member
      – Unrelated volunteer
Xenogeneic: Different species donor

---

phenotypically (albeit not genotypically) identical to those of the patient. Dependent upon the frequency of a patient's HLA alleles that make up the two haplotypes inherited from father and mother respectively, in a given population (see Table 3), the chances of finding such a donor may range from $1:100$ to $1:10^6$ or even less. Based on basic population genetics, it is clear that the probability of finding a donor is highest in a population of the same ethnic background as the patient.

Over the past decade considerable efforts have been made around the world to establish registries where HLA typing data of volunteers are listed in computer files, easily accessible for potential donor searches. Many of the registries, such as the

Anthony Nolan Appeal in Great Britain, owe their existence to the initiative of individuals searching for a donor for a family member; others, such as the National Marrow Donor Program in the U.S.A., are based on a broader organizational effort. Overall, there are currently HLA data on approximately one million potential donors stored in various files. Generally, serological typing data for class I antigens HLA-A and -B were entered first, but the number of individuals on whom class II data are stored as well is growing rapidly. The latter is important because this will shorten the search time.

Experience with unrelated volunteer marrow donors is still limited. However, currently more patients are being transplanted from unrelated than from HLA-nonidentical related donors. An initial informal search for an HLA-A and -B matched donor, for example, through the National Marrow Donor Program, can be carried out quickly and can be initiated by individual hematologists or oncologists without going through a transplant center. However, the fact that there is information on such an individual in the computer does not mean that a donor has been found. Firstly, it is possible that these potential donors are no longer available; they may have changed their mind (there is always some lag time before this is reflected in the computer) or for professional or private reasons are unable to respond. Even if they are willing and able to serve, it may take time to locate them. Secondly, additional typing for antigens not previously determined may have to be carried out. If by conventional techniques a match is confirmed, techniques such as isoelectric focusing (for HLA class I) and SSOP (as described below, for class II) are applied to further characterize identity or non-identity. These tests are currently considered a prerequisite since transplant results with donors mismatched at any level are inferior to results obtained with perfectly matched marrows. Two to six months or even more time may elapse before this work-up is complete, a transplant can be arranged, and a date for marrow harvest set.

Autologous Marrow

The current requirement for normal marrow status at the time of harvest largely limits autologous marrow transplantation to use as a "rescue" procedure for certain cancer patients undergoing intensive cytotoxic therapy. However, once gene transfer procedures become practical, autologous marrow transplantation may be applicable to certain inherited immunohematologic disorders (Table 3). When using autologous marrow, we are not truly dealing with a *transplant* procedure since no transfer to a different person is involved, but rather the *re-infusion* of previously aspirated marrow which one might term autoplantation.

The primary advantages of autologous marrow are that it is extensively available and that it lacks the immunologic complications of allogeneic marrow transplants – rejection and GVHD. Potential disadvantages include marrow abnormalities that would result in delayed marrow recovery assumed to be due to damage to the hemopoietic stem cell compartment or the microenvironment inflicted by prior cytotoxic therapy or stem cell damage due to flawed cryopreservation; also the absence of a "graft-vs.-leukemia" (allogeneic) effect, and the possibility of inadvertent reinfusion of occult clonogenic tumor cells that might cause relapse. The requirement for a normal (or nearly-normal) marrow at the time of harvest is a major disadvantage of autologous marrow transplants. This requirement excludes many patients with chronic lymphocytic leukemia and certain non-Hodgkin lymphomas who might otherwise be candidates for myeloablative therapy. Unfortunately, the diseases most responsive to escalated-dose therapy are also the diseases most likely to have marrow contamination with malignant cells. The most frequent cause of recurrence following autologous marrow transplantation, however, is not the reinfusion of such cells (in vitro failure) but rather failure of the conditioning regimen or other systemic therapies (in vivo failure), as indicated by experience in syngeneic marrow transplant recipients where relapse rates are high, even though normal marrow is transplanted. Therefore, the purging of malignant cells from autologous marrow, although likely important in certain diseases, is clearly futile if effective measures (including but not limited to conditioning) aimed at eradicating the disease. Nevertheless, some marrow purging is generally required; this is further discussed in II.2.

Recent studies suggest that not only marrow but also stem cells circulating in peripheral blood can be used for autologous transplantation, as previously shown in animal models. The use of peripheral stem cells may result in a faster hemopoietic recovery than achieved with marrow, particularly if these stem cells are "mobilized" by preceding administration of cytotoxic chemotherapy or recombinant hemopoietic growth factors. Some investigators speculate that the risk of infusing malignant cells into the patient may be lower with peripheral blood than with marrow stem cells.

Histocompatibility

Next to the patient's underlying disease the most important factor determining outcome after allogeneic transplantation appears to be the degree of histocompatibility with the marrow donor. The HLA antigens are encoded for by genes located on the short arm of chromosome 6. In addition, there are so-called minor, non-HLA histocompatibility antigens. It has been very difficult in man to further characterize the latter, and basically all transplants carried out to date have dealt with donor and recipient pairs characterized for HLA, but not for minor antigens. The inheritance of HLA genes follows a Mendelian pattern, i.e., every individual will have inherited one gene region, called a haplotype, from the father, and one from the mother. HLA antigens are highly polymorphic. By definition, however, there can be at most four haplotypes within each nuclear family (parents and children). Consequently, each patient who has a sibling has a theoretical chance of one in four that the sibling is HLA-identical (unless a crossover has occurred), and in fact ≈30–35% of Caucasian patients who have sisters or brothers are found to have an HLA-identical donor.

HLA identity is determined by using serological, cellular and molecular assays. Present HLA terminology is based on agreements reached at the Tenth International Histocompatibility Workshop. Histocompatibility typing should be carried out by an experienced laboratory, which has access to the latest typing reagents and uses the internationally accepted terminology. Generally, such laboratories will type patient and potential donor cells for HLA A, B, C, and DR, and possibly also DP and DQ, using alloantisera. In addition, cells will be set up against each other in a mixed leukocyte culture (MLC) to determine whether other antigens, referred to as HLA-D, not recognized by serological typing, lead to allogeneic stimulation of these cells as measured by radioactive thymidine uptake into replicating DNA. Occasionally patients and siblings have been typed and found to be completely identical, at least in appearance (phenotype), for all serologically determined antigens, yet the respective cells show mutual reactivity in MLC. Such a discrepancy is observed in less than 5% of sibling typings. Also, even if both serological typing and MLC results show identity, it is still possible that this is due to phenotypic rather than genotypic identity. This can occur, if the parents each express the same alleles on one of their two haplotypes. For example, both the father and mother may have HLA A2/B7 phenotypes, which are derived from different *genetic* backgrounds. Consequently, one of their children might have inherited the paternal A2/B7 haplotype, and one the maternal A2/B7 haplotype. Unless complete parent typing, ideally including additional antigens encoded for by genes on the short arm of chromosome 6 (e.g., complement factors), is available, a clear segregation of the genetic information cannot be determined, and occasionally it may not be possible to separate phenotypic from genotypic identity. Hence, whenever available, parents should be included in HLA typing studies. Occasionally typing of children may also be useful.

Recent development of molecular techniques and their application to HLA typing have refined our ability to characterize differences between patient and donor. The analysis of DNA extracted from cells by means of digestion with restriction enzymes and comparison of the size of the resulting fragments by Southern blotting, i.e., the determination of restriction fragment length polymorphism (RFLP), or hybridization of patient and donor DNA with oligonucleotides of known sequence capable of annealing with the complementary sequences at previously identified highly polymorphic DNA regions (sequence specific oligonucleotide probes, or SSOP), can identify even single base-pair difference. The decision as to who else in the family should be typed and at what level typing should be carried out must be arrived at after a discussion with an expert in an HLA laboratory, ideally at a marrow transplant facility.

Although most transplants carried out and reported to date have involved HLA-identical donors, the possibility of marrow transplantation should be considered even if no HLA-identical family member can be identified. The number of HLA-nonidentical transplants carried out at various centers is growing rapidly. Early results are encouraging, in that patients who are transplanted from a donor who differs for only one HLA antigen (HLA A, B, or D/DR) have a prognosis not significantly inferior to that observed with completely HLA-identical transplants. This is particularly true if patients are transplanted for a lymphohemopoietic malignancy while in chemotherapy-induced remission. Results become less convincing in patients transplanted while in relapse or for non-malignant conditions, such as severe aplastic anemia. Outcome becomes less encouraging as the extent of histoincompatibility increases, i.e., as two or even three antigenic regions (complete haplotype) are mismatched between donor and recipient. Problems include an increased incidence and severity of GVHD, failure of sustained engraftment, and infectious complications, both early and late after transplantation.

In some instances the requirements for HLA matching can be relaxed. For example, in a child with severe combined immunodeficiency, as pointed out earlier, haploidentical transplantation from father or mother, usually after T-cell depletion of the marrow, can be carried out successfully. In this setting, engraftment is often incomplete, i.e., only T lymphocytes may engraft, but this is all that is required in order to render these children immunocompetent. They do well utilizing their own hemopoietic system and B cells.

Table 6. Factors other than histocompatibility which affect donor selection

---
Donor/Patient sex match
Donor allosensitization
  (generally previous pregnancy in female donors)
Donor viral immunity
– Cytomegalovirus
– Hepatitis virus
– Human immunodeficiency virus
Donor age
ABO/Rh blood groups
Lymphocytotoxic antibodies in patient serum
Socioeconomic considerations
– Donor commitment
– Donor employment

Factors Other Than Histocompatibility Influencing Donor Selection

When choosing a donor, parameters other than histocompatibility also need to be taken into consideration (Table 6), and factors such as the potential donor's medical condition, sex, prior sensitization, the risks associated with anesthesia (during the marrow harvest), and psychological stability, including the donor's relationship to the patient, may be relevant Finally, patient age is of importance, since it appears that with syngeneic and autologous transplants a more advanced patient age (65 years and possibly even older) than with allogeneic transplants is still compatible with survival.

Since marrow aspiration is carried out on the anesthetized donor (general or, less frequently, epidural anesthesia), it is important to exclude the existence of any condition or illness that would increase the donor's anesthetic risk. This is of particular importance in female donors of childbearing age. If a female donor is being considered, a pregnancy test must be obtained. If a potential donor is found to be pregnant, ideally an alternative donor should be searched for. If no such alternative is available, the transplant may perhaps be delayed. In patients with certain diagnoses, e.g., chronic myelogenous leukemia or acute nonlymphoblastic leukemia in first remission, such an approach may be feasible. In other instances, for instance, advanced leukemia, this may not be an option. In such a situation, the potential risk to the pregnant woman and the fetus will have to be weighed against the potential benefit to the patient. This may be a difficult ethical decision; however, in some instances pregnant women have served as marrow donors without adverse effects to themselves or to the fetus.

Age is, similarly, a relative contraindication for marrow donation because of known increase in anesthetic risk with increasing age. Most transplant centers have excluded individuals more than 60 years of age from marrow donation. In all instances, however, it is important to evaluate potential donors individually, and even individuals more than 70 years of age have served uneventfully as allogeneic donors. While related donors as young as 2–3 months of age have donated marrow, the age of unrelated volunteer donors has generally been restricted to 18–50 years.

ABO incompatibility represents less of a problem in marrow transplantation than in renal transplantation. Blood group differences between donor and recipient may require manipulation or the marrow or isoagglutinin removal from the patient's plasma before marrow infusion (see II.2).

The effect of lymphocytotoxic antibodies on marrow engraftment is still controversial. However, in some situations, especially with HLA-nonidentical transplants, the presence of lymphocytotoxic antibodies directed at donor cells represents another risk factor for non-engraftment. These patients have generally been treated with plasmapheresis pretransplant to remove antibodies. In currently ongoing studies, attempts are being made to provide additional immunosuppression in the form of ATG or anti-T cell monoclonal antibody to assure engraftment.

There are data to suggest that sex differences may carry an increased risk of graft rejection in patients with aplastic anemia (male donor, female recipient) or may cause more GVHD (female donor, male recipient). Similarly, prior allosensitization, usually pregnancy in female donors and increased donor age have been found to increase the probability of GVHD.

There has always been concern that viruses may be transmitted from the donor to the patient, who may then be at high risk of developing a symptomatic infection because of transplant-related immunosuppression. If there is a choice between a CMV-positive and CMV-negative donor (all other factors being identical), the CMV-negative donor is preferable because the risk of CMV infection in the patient (particularly in the CMV-negative patient) is expected to be lower.

Since autologous transplantation circumvents transplant-related problems such as the development of GVHD, physicians may face the question of an autologous versus an allogeneic transplant if an HLA-identical family donor is available. This is further discussed in II.3.

Summary

While certain diagnoses, e.g., severe aplastic anemia or CML, clearly ask for an allogeneic (or syngeneic) donor, the decision is more difficult with diagnoses such as AML. While in patients with certain congenital disorders, CML and some other diagnoses transplantation offers the only change for cure, in patients with acute leukemia or malignant lymphoma this issue may be controversial. The decision in favor of transplantation, especially allogeneic transplantation, is made more easily in pediatric patients or young adults than in older patients. The decision making process should always involve an experienced transplant team.

References

Anasetti C, Amos D, Beatty PG, Appelbaum FR, Bensinger W, Buckner CD, Clift R, Doney K, Martin PJ, Mickelson E, Nisperos B, O'Quigley J, Ramberg R, Sanders JE, Stewart P, Storb R, Sullivan KM, Witherspoon RP, Thomas ED, Hansen JA (1989) Effect of HLA compatibility on engraftment of bone marrow transplants in patients with leukemia or lymphoma. N Engl J Med 320:197–204

Areman EM, Deeg HJ, Sacher RA (1992) Bone Marrow and Stem Cell Processing: A Manual of Current Techniques. F A Davis & Co. Philadelphia

Beatty PG, Dahlberg S, Mickelson EM, Nisperos B, Opelz G, Martin PJ, Hansen JA (1988) Probability of finding HLA-matched unrelated marrow donors. Transplantation 45:714–718

Blazar BR, Lasky LC, Perentesis JP, Watson KV, Steinberg SE, Filipovich AH, Orr HT, Ramsay NKC (1986) Successful donor cell engraftment in a recipient of bone marrow from a cadaveric donor. Blood 67:1655

Bortin MM, Advisory Committee (IBMTR), Buckner CD (1983) Seattle Marrow Transplant Team. Major complications of marrow harvesting for transplantation. Exp Hematol 11:916–921

Bowden RA, Slichter SJ, Sayers MH, Mori M, Cays MJ, Meyers JD (1991) Use of leukocyte-depleted platelets and cytomegalovirus-seronegative red blood cells for prevention of primary cytomegalovirus infection after marrow transplant. Blood 78:246–250

Buckner CD, Clift RA, Sanders JE, Stewart P, Bensinger WI, Doney KC, Sullivan KM, Witherspoon RP, Deeg HJ, Appelbaum FR, Storb R, Thomas ED (1984) Marrow harvesting from normal donors. Blood 64: 630–634

Fisher A, Durandy A, de Villartay JP, Vilmer E, Le Deist F, Gerota I, Griscelli C (1986) HLA- haploidentical bone marrow transplantation for severe combined immunodeficiency using E rosette fractionation and cyclosporine. Blood 67:444

Gingrich RD, Ginder GD, Goeken NE, Howe CWS, Wen BC, Hussey DH, Fyfe MA (1988) Allogeneic marrow grafting with partially mismatched, unrelated marrow donors. Blood 71:1375–1381

Hows JM, Yin JL, Marsh J, Swirsky D, Jones L, Apperley JF, James DCO, Smithers S, Batchelor JR, Goldman JM, Gordon-Smith EC (1986) Histocompatible unrelated volunteer donors compared with HLA nonidentical family donors in marrow transplantation for aplastic anemia and leukemia. Blood 68:1322–1328

Kersey JH, Weisdorf D, Nesbit ME, LeBien TW, Woods WG, McGlave PB, Kim T, Vallera DA, Goldman AI, Bostrom B, Hurd D, Ramsay NKC (1987) Comparison of autologous and allogeneic bone marrow transplantation for treatment of high-risk refractory acute lymphoblastic leukemia. N Engl J Med 317:461–467

Lonnqvist B, Ringden O, Wahren B, Gahrton G, Lundgren G (1984) Cytomegalovirus infection associated with and preceding chronic graft-versus-host disease. Transplantation 38:465–468

McGlave PB, Beatty P, Ash R, Hows JM (1990) Therapy for chronic myelogenous leukemia with unrelated donor bone marrow transplantation: Results in 102 cases. Blood 75:1728–1732

3. Preparation for Marrow Transplantation

Overview

This section deals with the logistics of readying a patient for marrow transplantation; the elements of this process are outlined in Table 7. Not all of these elements will be universally applicable, but will depend on diagnosis and type of marrow to be utilized. Since the use of normal marrow donor transplantation is often the standard, this approach will be used as a model; the elements are clearly different, to a degree, for autologous marrow transplant patients, and such will also be discussed.

Referral and Initial Consultation

Role of the Transplant Team

It is vital that frank communication between the Transplant Team and the patient, family and referring physician be established from the outset. This is especially important because marrow transplantation is associated with frequent morbidity and mortality, and few patients are fully aware of all potential adverse consequences when they are initially evaluated. Also, the Transplant Team member consulted should be capable of accurately discussing non-transplant treatment options in detail. If this is not the case, an appropriate consultation with other specialists should be obtained promptly to discuss such options.

Table 7. Patient preparation for marrow transplantation

A. Full discussion of marrow transplantation, including its rationale, risks and benefits with the patient, donor, other family and referring physician. Particular attention must be devoted to discussing alternative therapies and less obvious sequelae of marrow transplantation (e.g., growth retardation, chronic GVHD, sterility, second malignancy, etc.).
B. Complete medical history of both patient and donor, including:
   1. Unequivocal documentation of diagnosis
   2. Details of previous treatment, including cumulative doses of certain prior (especially cytotoxic) agents, as well as the level of response obtained
   3. Specific disease or treatment-related problems
   4. Co-morbid medical problems that might complicate or preclude transplantation
   5. Allergies, especially to commonly-used medications
   6. Transfusions, including number, type, results, reactions
   7. Psychologic assessment, with special attention to understanding of the procedure
C. Tumor staging studies for malignant diseases
   1. Bone marrow biopsy
   2. Central nervous system
   3. Sanctuary sites
   4. Others as required
D. Organ toxicity screening
   1. Pertinent history (see B2 and B3 above)
   2. Renal
      – Urinalysis
      – Serum creatinine
      – Creatinine clearance
   3. Hepatic
      – Liver function studies
   4. Pulmonary
      – Arterial blood gases
      – Pulmonary function studies
      – Diffusing capacity of carbon monoxide (DLCO)
   5. Cardiac
      – Left ventricular function evaluation
   6. Endocrine
      – Fasting blood sugar
      – Glucose tolerance test (optimal)
      – Thyroid function battery
      – Andrology (for sperm banking)
E. Histocompatibility testing for allogeneic and syngeneic marrow transplantation
   1. Serologic typing on patient and nuclear (or extended) family
   2. Mixed leukocyte culture (MLC) testing on the patient and prospective donor
   3. Molecular studies (may complement or replace MLC – and, eventually, serology)
F. Identification of marker of engraftment for allogeneic marrow transplantation
G. Transfusion support planning in all patients
   1. Evaluation of allosensitization status
   2. ABO typing of patient and donor
   3. Cytomegalovirus (CMV) status of patient and donor

Role of the Referring Physician

After the referring physician has given preliminary consideration to the patient's suitability for marrow transplantation (see I.1), contact with the Transplant Team is required to more fully assess the use of marrow transplantation.

The referring physician plays a key role in preparing a potential patient and donor for marrow transplantation. In addition to helping to assess the medical suitability of the procedure, the referring physician may be able to point out important non-medical considerations, (e.g., certain family interactions) that could have bearing on the case. Moreover, the physician may function as the patient's advocate in certain circumstances, especially when he/she has a large experience with alternative (i.e., non-transplant) therapies. If the referring physician and the Transplant Team decide to proceed with a formal evaluation, it is most helpful if the physician transmits to the Team the patient's complete medical records as well as initial histocompatibility data (although most Transplant Centers repeat these studies) – facsimile machines are invaluable in this regard. Also, the referring physician is usually able to facilitate the transfer of diagnostic materials for re-evaluation. In return, the referring physician should be kept fully informed of the results of the evaluation and the anticipated schedule of the procedure.

Depending on the resources available at the Transplant Center, the referral process may be expedited if the referring physician performs certain pre-transplant studies, including tumor staging, baseline organ toxicity determinations, and placement of an indwelling central venous catheter. A medical evaluation of the donor may also be useful in some cases.

The referring physician will play an important role in the patient's continuing care after discharge from the Transplant Center. The policy of close communication noted above, established soon after the patient's initial evaluation, will allow optimal post-transplant management.

Discussion with the Patient

When patients are first evaluated by the Transplant Team, they may have widely varying amounts of information and perceptions regarding marrow transplantation. In any case, the key aspects of transplantation should be discussed fully with the patient and their family. Repetition and complete documentation of such discussions are necessary. Despite this requirement, the first contact should be simple and straightforward as the patient's ability to absorb large quantities of unfamiliar information during an initial (and often stressful) visit is often limited.

In addition to further discussions, pamphlets and other resource materials are helpful in imparting information to the patient; of particular benefit is a videocassette describing the marrow transplant procedure that the patient may borrow, if such is available. Patients and families often appreciate being given a tour of the Transplant Unit prior to admission and the opportunity to meet other members of its staff (especially nursing personnel) during their initial visit.

Some prospective patients also request that they be allowed to meet with patients who have had transplants. In this matter, caution should be exercised – both to ensure patient confidentiality and to avoid bias. (For example, there is an obvious tendency to arrange a meeting with a patient whose post-transplant course was relatively uncomplicated, perhaps obscuring the negative aspects of the procedure.) To a degree, these problems may be circumvented by providing access to a volunteer support group of former bone marrow transplant patients.

The initial discussion may begin with a review of the patient's diagnosis and current disease status, as well as an anticipation of the natural history of the underlying disease. The rationale for considering marrow transplantation, both in general and for the patient's specific disease in particular, should follow. The prognosis after marrow transplantation must be compared in detail with that for other treatment options; this aspect is of particular importance for patients in whom other potentially-curative treatment options exist (for instance, patients with acute leukemia in an initial remission who are potentially curable with additional chemotherapy alone). Moreover, certain less obvious points should be detailed; for example, an acute leukemia patient may have been a reasonable candidate for transplantation soon after first achieving an initial complete remission, but be much less so after a year of continuous remission. Also, although the chief reason for considering a marrow transplant is almost always the possibility of cure, some patients arrive with the misconception that marrow transplantation is invariably curative; this idea must be dispelled. If entry onto a research study is planned, the prospective patient should be informed at this time.

The immediate and delayed toxicities of marrow transplantation must be detailed; the period of pancytopenia and hospitalization after the transplant, especially in a patient who has previously undergone intensive chemotherapy, is only the most obvious. The other major complications (e.g., graft failure, regimen-related toxicity, graft-vs-host disease [GVHD] and various infections) must be discussed fully.

Although fatal toxicities are more obvious, it is also important to discuss the possibility of persistent debilities of a non-fatal nature, especially those related to chronic GVHD, growth retardation, sterility and aseptic necrosis of weight-bearing joints; in particular, some patients who develop these problems, especially severe and unremitting chronic GVHD, understandably may become quite embittered – even if they have been cured of an otherwise-fatal illness. Other late complications should also be discussed, even if they are poorly defined. The possibility of an increased risk of second malignancy must be mentioned. Although many male patients with previously-treated malignancy may be sterile before conditioning, the option of sperm banking should be discussed. Finally, it should be noted that the number of transplant patients followed for more than 10–15 years is relatively small, and as-yet-unrecognized late complications may arise.

Of course, patients frequently need some idea of their chances for cure. This is a potentially difficult area; for instance, if one's own institutional results are markedly different from those of a more general experience (e.g., the International

Bone Marrow Transplant Registry [IBMTR]), which should be provided? While there is no simple answer, one approach is to provide data from a large experience (e.g., the IBMTR) but stress that these are only estimations, and that particular features of the patient or their treatment may alter these results. Again, if patients are being entered into research studies, the investigational nature of same should be addressed.

It is important to guard against the possibility that the enthusiasm of a member of the Transplant Team might subtly influence a patient to accept a transplant rather than more conventional therapy. Such acceptance of marrow transplantation on less than reasonable grounds is particularly undesirable since marrow transplantation is still plagued by high intrinsic morbidity and (more variably) mortality rates, to say nothing of expense.

When informed consent is obtained, it should be fully documented and witnessed; the patient should be given ample opportunity for questions and – if necessary – withdrawal. In this regard, some patients voice troubling thoughts such as "What choice do I have?" or "I have nothing to lose." Although these statements may indeed hold true regarding cure, the option of alternative therapy (or occasionally even no further therapy) must always be kept open, and some discussion should take place to the effect that early transplant-related mortality may involve a greater degree of trauma for patient and family compared with a quieter, more fully palliated end. Obviously, this delicate area must be handled with considerable sensitivity to the emotional impact of the issues involved.

Discussion with the Potential Donor

Most potential donors are eager to participate but may have concerns which they may be reluctant to voice (e.g., fear of anesthesia or needles) or have a history of social habits with major potential consequences to the outcome of the transplant (e.g., certain patterns of sexual behavior or intravenous drug use that may predispose to human immunodeficiency virus [HIV] infection). Potential donors must be asked specifically about these matters, as well as about their concerns regarding the procedure itself. It should be noted that some such discussions should take place without the patient or other family members being present, and donors should (in a discreet manner) be offered this option.

Although donors generally desire to assist the patient, it is likely that in many cases a potential donor may not exercise any real choice regarding participation in the transplant, as it has been taken for granted that he or she will donate marrow. Of course, such an assumption should not be made; a potential donor who is fully informed and truly does not wish to donate marrow should be supported in this decision.

Finally, a preliminary psychological assessment of the potential donor should be performed, as the stress associated with the procedure may exacerbate a chronic psychological condition. At worst, a potential donor could withdraw consent and refuse to donate at a critical time; more commonly, a donor may take on an inappropriate burden of guilt for post-transplant complications (especially graft failure or GVHD). When anything but the mildest psychologic dysfunction is suspected in the preliminary assessment, consultation with a psychiatrist is recommended.

Medical Evaluation

Obviously, a complete evaluation, beginning with a history and physical exam, is required on the patient. The following points deserve special emphasis.

Confirmation of Diagnosis and Disease Status

Diagnosis

This point appears to be self-evident. However, some patients arrive at the Transplant Center with no evidence of disease (e.g., acute leukemia patients in remission) and prompt confirmation is mandatory in these and all other cases. Ideally, tissues obtained from previous diagnostic studies should be reviewed by a pathologist who works closely with the Transplant Team. If any questions arise, additional specimens from previous tissue sections or repeat biopsy procedures may be required; even a seemingly minor discrepancy (e.g., a misclassification of the type or disease status of acute leukemia) may be important, as some Transplant Centers have different treatment regimens for these conditions.

Disease Status

For patients who have active malignant disease, it is important to know the sites and extent of disease. This will not only impact on prognosis but will also be important regarding the use of adjunctive special therapies (e.g., local radiotherapy to nodes obstructing vital structures or to testicular tumors, intrathecal or intraventricular chemotherapy for malignant meningeal deposits, etc.). In brief, thorough restaging (often including repeat biopsy) is recommended.

There are at least two reasons to document the activity and extent of a malignant disease immediately before transplantation. First, active disease may be an indication for therapy in addition to the conditioning regimen, or perhaps for an altered conditioning regimen. Second, the presence of advanced disease is usually an important negative prognostic factor for the outcome of marrow transplantation, and detection of such may bring about the use of different therapeutic components – or even cancellation of the procedure.

Such evaluations are not generic to marrow transplantation and will differ with various diseases. Therefore, specific required studies are not listed. In general, however, previous sites of disease should again be evaluated, as well as others likely to be involved subclinically. Biopsy should be obtained as soon as possible if the findings might have influence the decision to transplant or result in a major change in therapy.

For autologous marrow transplantation, a recent (i.e., within approximately 2 weeks) bone marrow aspirate and biopsy is required both to document that marrow is histologically normal (or, in the rare case in which such is not required, that a satisfactory specimen is present) and to ensure that the marrow can be aspirated easily; this is especially important in patients with marrow-based malignancies and fibrosis and in those with a prior history of cytotoxic therapy, especially pelvic radiotherapy. More sophisticated studies (e.g., the use of molecular methods such as the polymerase chain reaction) to assess "minimal residual disease" may achieve importance in the future but are not routinely utilized at present.

Previous Treatment

This point is important for two reasons. Firstly, the level of response to prior therapy (e.g., the history of a previous remission with conventional antileukemic chemotherapy) may provide important information about prognosis after transplantation or dictate changes in the transplant regimen – in particular, patients with chemotherapy-resistant malignancy are poor candidates for marrow transplantation. Secondly, the potential cumulative toxicity from such therapy might pose excessive hazards after transplantation; although difficult to quantitate, in general the more extensive the previous treatment, the greater the post-transplant toxicity expected. The Transplant Team needs to be aware, for example, of the cumulative doses received of agents that often produce non-hematologic toxicity (e.g., anthracyclines, cisplatin, bleomycin and radiation), as well as any evidence of existing toxicity from these agents (see below).

Co-Morbid Medical Problems

A careful history and subsequent evaluation concerning this aspect should be performed. Specifically, a previous history of cardiac, renal, endocrine or hepatic disease must be solicited, as underlying disease in these organs may complicate transplantation.

Organ Toxicity Screening

Patients should not have impairment of any organ system that would might jeopardize an otherwise-successful transplant. It is important to emphasize that pre-transplant impairment may be subclinical or subtle, only to become manifest after the "stress" of the conditioning regimen or transplant. Therefore, systematic evaluation of liver, kidney, lung, heart and perhaps certain endocrine gland functions should be performed.

More specifically, the history and physical examination of the patient are important, especially focusing upon the prior therapy history and serious co-morbid conditions that may produce a compromised organ (e.g., extensive anthracycline therapy and cardiac disease). In addition to routine hepatic and renal serum assays, a creatinine clearance and a complete battery of pulmonary function tests are desirable. However, there are certain problems with some screening tests: for example, assays of cardiac left ventricular function are of low yield in patients with a negative cardiac history, and any or all of these tests may not reliably detect subclinical dysfunction.

Allergies

Although a history of documented or probable allergies is part of the routine examination, special attention should be directed to those agents which the patient may receive peri-transplant, specifically allopurinol, trimethoprim-sulfamethoxazole, and β-lactam antibiotics.

Evaluation of Infection Potential

It is important to be aware of previous infections that may be quiescent but which may be reactivated during the severe immunosuppression following the conditioning regimen. Examples include tuberculosis, aspergillosis and diseases related to herpes viruses. Prophylaxis (e.g., with antubercular drugs, amphotericin B or acyclovir) may be indicated. Some infections (e.g., HIV) may actually contraindicate transplantation.

It should be mentioned here that the medical evaluation of the donor is also important in this regard. Transmission of donor infections such as malaria, hepatitis B or HIV has been reported. Hepatitis C infection of the donor is currently considered by some investigators to be a relative (but not an absolute) contraindication to using such a donor.

Given the effectiveness of the simple modality of CMV-negative transfusions in preventing serious CMV infections, it is critical to determine the CMV status of the patient and donor. If the patient is negative, seronegative donors are strongly preferred, but if a seropositive donor is used, the prophylactic use of ganciclovir in the recipient has dramatically reduced clinically relevant CMV disease.

Management of existing infections in the patient pre-transplant is discussed below.

Transfusions

Specifics concerning the number, type, result and reactions to previous transfusions with all blood components must be obtained, as this information could influence the type of conditioning required, especially for patients with severe aplastic anemia. Issues concerning transfusion support peri-transplant are discussed below.

It is most important to delineate pre-transplant the extent of allosensitization, a condition that may render platelet transfusions (which are required until the transplant is fully functional) ineffective. Transplantation should be undertaken only after careful consideration if severe allosensitization is documented.

Psychologic Assessment

Some centers perform routine psychologic screening of all patients. This may be desirable, but is probably unneccessary unless a previous history of psychologic instability (or an actual psychiatric diagnosis) is known or suspected. In such cases, continuation of established liaisons between the patient and a psychiatrist or psychologist may be helpful.

Of course, most patients considering marrow transplantation have an appropriate degree of anxiety. However, it is necessary to distinguish such patients from others who enter the marrow transplantation procedure with the anxiety produced by a psychiatric diagnosis that precludes incomplete understanding of the procedure or the ability to give informed consent. If transplanted, patients in the latter group may be expected to respond poorly to information concerning unexpected complications and related requests for unexpected invasive procedures (e.g., open lung biopsy for interstitial pneumonitis). Obviously, identifying such patients and obtaining appropriate consultation pre-transplant is vital.

Donor Preference

Autologous Versus Allogeneic Marrow

Although autologous marrow transplants are most often considered in the context of patients without histocompatible donors, there are circumstances in which using autologous marrow may be preferable to using allogeneic marrow.

In general, autotransplants are preferred in older patients, regardless of the presence of suitable donors. Also, for most malignant solid tumors (perhaps excluding neuroblastoma), the probability of cure is low with current conditioning regimens and the risks associated with allogeneic marrow transplantation do not appear to routinely justify the use of this modality.

Of course, not all patients are eligible for both types of transplant, due to relatively advanced age, histocompatibility limitations, marrow contamination with malignant cells or other major treatment-related complications such as persistent aplasia, myelodysplasia, and myelofibrosis.

More difficult is the question of allogeneic versus autologous transplantation in a patient eligible for either. Several studies have been published (for acute lymphoblastic leukemia and malignant lymphoma) in which these two types of marrow were compared, albeit in a non-randomized fashion. Results in terms of disease-free survival have been similar, with a higher risk of recurrence in the autologous patients offset by a higher rate of non-relapse mortality in the allograft patients. Stated another way, the benefits of a graft-versus-leukemia/lymphoma effect were offset by GVHD. (These specific expectations may be useful in a particular patient: for instance, patients with a relatively lower risk of surviving GVHD and of subsequent recurrence may best be treated with an autotransplant, while those more likely to survive GVHD but with a higher risk of recurrence should be considered for an allogeneic transplant preferentially.)

However, the above comparative results, while interesting, should be interpreted with caution: one should not merely assume that either source of marrow may be used in a case in which either is possible. For instance, allogeneic marrow transplantation is more-or-less standard therapy in patients with acute myelogenous leukemia in first complete remission under the age of 50 years (and more so <30 years), and autologous transplantation in such patients is more controversial. Conversely, autologous marrow transplantation is the more popular for certain Hodgkin's disease and non-Hodgkin's lymphoma patients, although it must be emphasized that definitive comparative data are unavailable. While comparative trials might be definitive, the difficulty in performing them is not to be underestimated, and such trials may not be performed.

Normal Donors

Due to the paucity of complications, syngeneic transplants are virtually always preferred, but this is of course a very rare option. Also, due to the lack of the graft-vs-leukemia/lymphoma effect noted above, the probability of relapse may be higher; it is conceivable (although unlikely) that a syngeneic donor would not be chosen if the risk of relapse were very high. Although in many instances an HLA-identical related donor is unavailable, the opposite situation may arise, in which more than one histocompatible donor will be identified. In this situation, the following selection criteria, approximately in the order listed, may be applied:

a) Donor consent, as well as donor medical and psychologic health. These considerations are usually obvious, but the issue of consent is particularly important (for a more thorough discussion, see I.2). While donor age should probably not routinely exceed 60–65 years, this is an infrequent consideration for related donors, since most allogeneic marrow transplants are performed between siblings who are roughly of similar age – usually younger than 60 years. Conversely, this situation may arise more often with "mismatched" related and unrelated donors. In any case, there is no consistent correlation between donor age and post-transplant complications, although the probability of GVHD will likely be higher with older donors.

b) CMV serologic status. If the patient is seronegative for CMV (i.e., has not been exposed to the virus previously), donors who are also seronegative for CMV are preferred.

c) Donor sex. Sex matching, and especially the avoidance of a parous (allosensitized) female donor for a male recipient, is preferable as this situation is associated with a greater probability of GVHD.

d) ABO blood type. If all other factors are equal, major ABO mismatches should be avoided since this occurrence complicates (albeit slightly) the transplant procedure technically (see below).

Histocompatibility Evaluation

Allogeneic Transplantation

When a patient is referred to a Transplant Center, histocompatibility testing of the HLA complex for the HLA-A, -B, -D/-DR alleles of the patient and (at least some) family members will often have been performed. If HLA typing has not been performed, or if, in the assessment of the Transplant Team, there is any question about its accuracy, tissue typing should be repeated at the Transplant Center. (As noted above, most centers prefer to repeat HLA typing in all patients.) Furthermore, it may be necessary to perform such typing in additional family members, especially parents and children, to delineate genotypic as opposed to phenotypic matching or to identify an alternative donor.

A member of the Transplant Team should be consulted concerning the timing or other specifics of the HLA testing whenever any question exists.

Identification of a Marker of Engraftment

For allogeneic marrow transplantation, identifying an informative marker of engraftment is highly desirable. Sex chromosome in cytogenetic analysis, erythrocyte phenotypic differences or DNA polymorphic sequences may be used. For "mismatched" transplants, HLA typing may be used.

Autologous Transplantation

Except for considerations of HLA-matched platelet transfusion support (as discussed below), histocompatibility testing is not routinely required in the autologous marrow transplantation setting.

Management of Existing Pre-Transplant Infections

(This subject is discussed more fully in III.4.) Patients with active or inadequately treated infections should be identified and started on appropriate therapy. While such infections should generally be resolved before conditioning begins, there are instances in which infections cannot be expected to improve without a successful graft. For example, for some patients with severe neutropenia due to an otherwise-untreatable underlying disease (such as severe aplastic anemia or certain cases of leukemia), only successful marrow transplantation would increase the neutrophil count. In these cases marrow transplantation should be expedited in order not to further extend the period of pancytopenia.

Transfusion Support

Certain problems (e.g., severe pre-transplant allosensitization or the presence of an unusual blood type) require special consideration from apheresis units and blood banks. In addition, patients who receive a marrow transplant from a donor with an incompatible major red blood cell group require special manipulations to avoid hemolysis with the marrow reinfusion and in the immediate post-transplant period (see II.2).

Ideally, several related or volunteer unrelated blood donors, HLA-matched with the patient, should be available for all transplant patients, but especially allosensitized patients (as discussed above).

Erythrocyte Support Problems

The need to support patients with red blood cells of an infrequent phenotype is not unique to marrow transplantation. Given adequate notice, blood banking facilities can usually deal with these problems by stockpiling a supply of frozen blood or via exchange with other blood centers, if necessary.

ABO-Incompatible Marrow Transplants

The problems with ABO− incompatible marrow infusion relate primarily to hemolysis. There is no strong evidence that even major incompatibilities adversely affect engraftment, GVHD or survival. The special precautions required in patients who receive ABO-incompatible marrow include the prevention of hemolysis with the procedure and the provision of appropriate changes in transfusion support post-transplant. Several methods to overcome hemolysis have been employed. In case of a major ABO mismatch (in which the patient has iso-agglutinins against the donor), plasmapheresis, or immuno-absorbent columns can be used to decrease the patient's isohemagglutinin titer. In addition, appropriate separation of the incompatible erythrocytes from donor marrow ex vivo will reduce the probability of a severe reaction. In case of a minor ABO mismatch (in which the donor has isoagglutinins against the patient), simple plasma removal from the donor marrow is sufficient. Post-transplant transfusion support can be managed by selecting blood components that avoid incompatible red cells and plasma. In any case, notification of the blood bank or apheresis staff during the planning stage of transplantation is vital.

Points of Emphasis

In some cases, preparation for transplantation is not urgent. In other circumstances, however, the need for prompt transplantation may necessitate compression of the usual preparation time. In either situation, one must take care to ensure that the evaluation is meticulous, and that the patient (and donor) have had sufficient time and information to arrive at the decision to proceed with a marrow transplant.

References

Andrykowski MA, Altmaier EM, Barnett RL, Otis ML, Gingrich R, Henslee-Downey PJ (1990) The quality of life in adult survivors of allogeneic bone marrow transplantation. Transplantation 50:399

Appelbaum FR, Sullivan KM, Buckner CD, Clift RA, Deeg HJ, Fefer A, Hill R, Mortimer J, Neiman PE, Sanders JE, Singer J, Stewart P, Storb R, Thomas ED (1987) Treatment of malignant lymphoma in 100 patients with chemotherapy, total body irradiation, and marrow transplantation. J Clin Oncol 5:1340

Bearman SI, Appelbaum FR, Back A, Petersen FB, Buckner CD, Sullivan KM, Schoch HG, Fisher LD, Thomas ED (1989) Regimen-related toxicity and early posttransplant survival in patients undergoing marrow transplantation for lymphoma. J Clin Oncol 7:1288

Bearman SI, Appelbaum FR, Buckner CD, Petersen FB, Fisher LD, Clift RA, Thomas ED (1988) Regimen-related toxicity in patients undergoing bone marrow transplantation. J Clin Oncol 6:1562

Beatty PG, Clift RA, Mickelson EM, Nisperos BB, Flournoy N, Martin PJ, Sanders JE, Stewart P, Buckner CD, Storb R, Thomas ED, Hansen JA (1985) Marrow transplantation from related donors other than HLA-identical siblings. N Engl J Med 313:765

Brack G, LaClave L, Blix S (1988) The psychological aspects of bone marrow transplant: A staff's perspective. Cancer Nurs 11:221

Crossreacting groups of HLA-A and B antigens. (1987) Tissue Typing Reference Manual (edition 2), South-Eastern Organ Procurement Foundation, Richmond, Virginia: p. 4.14

Deeg HJ (1990) Delayed complications and long-term effects after bone marrow transplantation. Hematol Oncol Clin North Am 4:641

Dermatis H, Lesko LM (1991) Psychosocial correlates of physician-patient communication at time of informed consent for bone marrow transplantation. Cancer Invest 9:621

Futterman AD, Wellisch DK (1990) Psychodynamic themes of bone marrow transplantation. When I becomes thou. Hematol Oncol Clin North Am 4:699

Hinterberger-Fischer M, Kier P, Kalhs P, Marosi C, Geissler K, Schwarzinger I, Pabinger I, Huber J, Spona J, Kolbabek H, Koren H, Muller G, Hawliczek R, Lechner K, Hayek-Rosenmayr A, Hinterberger W (1991) Fertility, pregnancies and offspring complications after bone marrow transplantation. Bone Marrow Transplant 7:5

Hows JM, Bradley BA (1990) The use of unrelated marrow donors for transplantation. Br J Haematol 76:1

Jones RJ, Ambinder RF, Piantadosi S, Santos GW (1991) Evidence of a graft-versus-lymphoma effect associated with allogeneic bone marrow transplantation. Blood 77:649

Kersey JH, Weisdorf D, Nesbit ME, LeBien TW, Woods WG, McGlave PB, Kim T, Vallera DA, Goldman AI, Bostrom B, Hurd D, Ramsay NKC (1987) Comparison of autologous and allogeneic bone marrow transplantation for treatment of high-risk refractory acute lymphoblastic leukemia. N Engl J Med 317:461

Lasky LC, Warkiniin PI, Kersey JH, Ramsay NKC, McGlave PB, McCullough J (1983) Hemotherapy in patients undergoing blood group incompatible bone marrow transplantation. Transfusion 23:277

Phillips GL (1992) Autologous bone marrow transplantation for hematologic malignancy. Drug Resistance as a Biochemical Target in Cancer Chemotherapy, Tsuruo T, Ogawa M, Carter WK (eds), Academic Press, San Diego, CA:295

Singer DA, Donnelly MB, Messerschmidt GL (1990) Informed consent for bone marrow transplantation: Identification of relevant information by referring physicians. Bone Marrow Transplant 6:431

Slichter SJ (1988) Transfusion and bone marrow transplantation. Transfusion Med Rev 2:1

Wingard JR, Curbow B, Baker F, Piantadosi S (1991) Health, functional status, and employment of adult survivors of bone marrow transplantation. Ann Intern Med 114:113

Wingard JR, Plotnick LP, Freemer CS, Zahurak M, Piantadosi S, Miller DF, Vriesendorp HM, Yeager AM, Santos GW (1992) Growth in children after bone marrow transplantation: Busulfan plus cyclophosphamide versus cyclophosphamide plus total body irradiation. Blood 79:1068

Wolcott DL, Wellisch DK, Fawzy FI, Landsverk J (1986) Adaptation of adult bone marrow transplant recipient long-term survivors. Transplantation 41:478

Wolcott DL, Wellisch DK, Fawzy FI, Landsverk J (1986) Psychological adjustment of adult bone marrow transplant donors whose recipient survives. Transplantation 41:484

4. Cost and Availability of Transplantation

Bone marrow transplantation is a complex and expensive procedure. Estimates provided by different transplant centers in the USA, for example, range from $150,000 to $250,000, about DM 200,000 in Germany and about $100,000 in Canada. The cost may vary from country to country and the "visible" expenses may depend upon the health care system by which the patient is covered. Regardless, however, expenses incurred with marrow transplantation fall into the category of "catastrophic illness" that patients are generally not able to pay out of pocket. In some economically weak countries, it may not be possible to carry out transplants routinely even though the technology is available. The actual cost will depend upon a patient's hospital course, since it is the hospitalization that accounts for the major fraction of the total bill. A major reduction of costs may be necessary to make transplantation more widely available.

When marrow transplantation was first used in the early 70s', research funds were often available to institutions carrying out marrow transplantation. As more and more marrow transplants were carried out, and the success rate improved, insurance carriers were called upon with increasing frequency to cover the cost. Certain diseases such as acquired severe aplastic anemia or inherited disorders such as SCID have been universally accepted as indications for marrow transplantation and are generally covered by insurance policies in many countries. Conversely, solid tumors and autologous transplants, are more controversial and often considered experimental by insurance carriers. An important consideration in addition to the diagnosis may be the disease phase or stage: should a transplant be carried out in a patient who has only a 5% chance of being cured? How can criteria be established? Who will make the decision? Although many investigators feel that for certain disease categories and patient groups, marrow transplantation may offer the best prognosis, a true consensus has not been reached.

It has been argued that these questions would be dealt with more easily in countries with a national health care system (e.g., England, Canada) or a comparable program. Experience in those countries, however, also reveals problems: although every patient may have the same chance to be transplanted, the system may determine which indications are acceptable and which ones are not. The increase in the number of available transplant beds has been slow due to a reluctance to invest heavily in this field. With the current interest in marrow transplantation in patients with carcinoma of the breast projections are such that the existing system could not support application of this modality to all candidates, both in regards to bed capacity and financial resources. Regardless of the system, the cost of bone marrow transplantation is high and the cost-benefit ratio increases as more high risk patients are being transplanted. One task for those working in the field is, therefore, to further improve the approach so that transplants can be carried out with greater success, with less toxicity and at a lower cost. Great hopes have been placed on hemopoietic growth factors which are now available in recombinant form.

It will be important, for any patient in whom marrow transplantation is considered, to discuss these plans with their respective insurance companies. It is helpful to have this information available at the time when a patient presents to a marrow transplant center. In the setting of allogeneic marrow transplantation, insurance carriers have usually been willing to pay for expenses incurred by the bone marrow donor, i.e., cost of short term hospitalization, anesthesia, time in the operating room, and brief post operative care. It should, however, also be noted that bone marrow donation will usually mean that the donor is away from work at least for a few days, and possibly for several weeks if he or she is required to serve as a platelet donor after transplantation. It is helpful to discuss this early on with the donor's employer in order to avoid unpleasant surprises later.

If no suitable donor can be identified within the family, and an unrelated donor search is initiated additional costs arise. With a search through national and especially international donor banks patients may incur expenses of the search and additional HLA typing work which may be reimbursed only later or occasionally not at all.

Finally, even after a transplant has been carried out successfully, the patient may not be able to return to work immediately and may be without work-related income for months or years. This experience may represent not only extraordinary financial problems but may also result in severe psychological stress and intrafamilial tension.

References

Trigg ME (1986) The decision in pediatrics to go ahead with bone marrow transplant for a pediatric malignancy. Bone Marrow Transplantation 1:111

Vaughan WP, Purtilo RD, Butler CD, Armitage JO (1986) Ethical and financial issues in autologous marrow transplantation: a symposium sponsored by the University of Nebraska Medical Center (editorial). Ann Int Med 105:134

Watson JG, Clink HM, Powles RL, Jameson B, Kay HEM, Lumley H (1981) Acute myeloid leukaemia: comparison of support required during initial induction of remission and marrow transplantation in first remission. The Lancet, II:957

Welch HG, Larson EB (1989) Cost effectiveness of bone marrow transplantation in acute nonlymphocytic leukemia. N Engl J Med 321:807–812

Woolhandler S, Himmelstein DU, Labar B, Lang S (1987) Transplanted technology: Third world options and first world science. N Engl J Med 317:504–506

II. Transplant Procedure

1. Conditioning Regimens

General Considerations

Shortly before the infusion of marrow, patients are generally given a course of dose-intensive chemotherapy, often with the addition of total body irradiation (TBI). This treatment is known as the conditioning (or preparative) regimen and is usually assumed to be myeloablative, although this is not always the case. At least in theory, different conditioning regimens may be preferred for different diseases or chosen based upon the source of marrow used for transplantation; in practice, one of several basic regimens is usually used with relatively few major, but fairly frequent minor alterations – a practice that contributes to the difficulty in comparing the efficacy and toxicity of various regimens.

Conditioning is generally considered to have two functions: immunosuppression and the removal of unwanted (usually malignant) cell populations. Agents with antineoplastic activity also may be used to remove an abnormal (albeit benign) cell population, as is the case in thalassemia. Agents frequently used in current conditioning regimens are listed in Table 8, according to their putative primary function – predominantly either immunosuppressive or antineoplastic. However, it should be noted that although this separation of function is useful in theory, it is an oversimplification, as there is considerable overlap and certain agents or modalities (e.g., TBI) are very potent in both regards.

Single-agent therapy is not widely used for conditioning, except in previously-untransfused aplastic anemia patients in whom cyclophosphamide alone at a cumulative dose of 200 mg/kg is considered the treatment of choice. Multiple agents are used because tolerable doses of most single agents

Table 8. Conditioning regimen components used in near-maximal doses[a]

Agents used primarily for immunosuppression
- Anti-thymocyte globulin (or variants)
- Cyclophosphamide
- Total lymphoid irradiation (TLI)

Agents used primarily for antineoplastic effects
- Busulfan
- Carmustine
- Cytarabine
- Etoposide
- Carboplatin
- Diaziquone

Agents used for both purposes
- Total body irradiation (TBI)
- Melphalan
- ThioTEPA

[a] Note: Other agents, especially those in which substantial dose escalation is impractical (e.g., daunorubicin, cisplatin, etc.) are not included in this compilation, even though they may be used in various conditioning regimens.

(other than TBI or perhaps melphalan) provide only marginal immunosuppression in other circumstances; multiple agents are also deemed necessary for optimal antineoplastic effects. These considerations have led to the construction of widely used two-agent regimens with each component given in escalated, often near-maximal single agent doses. Examples include cyclophosphamide plus TBI (CY + TBI) and busulfan plus cyclophosphamide (BUCY); details of administration are outlined in Tables 9, 10 and 11. Such regimens provide satisfactory immunosuppression for histocompatible allogeneic grafts, and acceptable if not wholly satisfactory antineoplastic effects – providing they are used in an early (preferably first) remission or stable phase. As with non-transplant antineoplastic therapies, relapse rates generally rise dramatically with more advanced disease and in situations in which a "graft-versus-tumor" effect is not present, notably syngeneic and autologous marrow transplantation.

While a further increase in the number of such agents would be expected to enhance antitumor effects, this approach

Table 9. Cyclophosphamide plus total body irradiation regimens in common use

Agent	Daily dose	Schedule	Total dose
A. Cyclophosphamide	60 mg/kg	Daily × 2 (days -5, -4)	120 mg/kg
Fractionated TBI	200 cGy	Twice daily × 3 (days -3, -2, -1)	1200 cGy
B. Cyclophosphamide	60 mg/kg	Daily × 2 (days -8, -7)	120 mg/kg
Fractionated TBI	200 cGy	Daily × 6 (days -6, -5, -4, -3, -2, -1)	1200 cGy
C. Cyclophosphamide	50 mg/kg	Daily × 4 (days -8, -7, -6, -5)	200 mg/kg
Fractionated TBI	300 cGy	Daily × 4 (days -4, -3, -2, -1)	1200[a] cGy
D. Fractionated TBI	360 cGy	Thrice daily × 3 (days -7, -6, -5), twice daily × 1 (day -4)	
Cyclophosphamide	60 mg/kg	Daily × 2 (days -3, -2)[b]	120 mg/kg

[a] Lung shielding after 900 cGy.
[b] Includes additional radiotherapy (i.e., electron boost) to chest wall and testes.

Table 10. Major chemoradiotherapy variants using drugs other than cyclophosphamide

Agent	Daily dose	Schedule	Total dose
A. Cytarabine	3 gm/m^2	q12h × 6 days (days -9 to -4)	36 g/m^2
Fractionated TBI	200 cGy	bid × 3 days (days -3 to -1)	1200 cGy
B. Fractionated TBI[a]	120 cGy	tid × 3 days (days -7 to -5)	1320 cGy
Etoposide	60 mg/kg	Daily × 1 (day -3)	60 g/kg

[a] Combined with lung shielding and boost electron therapy to the chest and testes.

has proven difficult if all agents are used in maximal doses, primarily because current conditioning regimens have a marginal therapeutic index that usually narrows with the addition of more agents or higher doses of the components. For example, regimens using high-dose etoposide or cytarabine instead of cyclophosphamide would be better tolerated than those including these agents plus cyclophosphamide. An alternative approach, in which other agents are added in submaximal doses (such as the variants of the "BACT" regimen described below, in which more-or-less conventional doses of carmustine [BCNU], cytarabine [arabinosyl cytosine] and thioguanine are used with near-maximal doses of cyclophosphamide), has not been used very widely in the construction of conditioning regimens, although more recently anthracyclines (in conventional dose) have been used in conditioning regimens for leukemia.

Detailed Requirements of the Conditioning Regimen

Immunosuppression

In allogeneic marrow transplants, suppression of the host-versus-graft reaction is required for stable engraftment. As discussed above, certain congenital immunodeficiency syndromes (e.g., severe combined immunodeficiency disease, SCID) are exceptions, as the intrinsic immune defect abrogates this requirement. Immunosuppression is generally not needed in

Table 11. Busulfan plus cyclophosphamide regimens in common use

Agent	Daily dose	Schedule	Total dose
A. Busulfan	4 mg/kg	q6h × 16 (days -9 to -6)	16 mg/kg
Cyclophosphamide	50 mg/kg	Daily × 4 (days -5 to -2)	200 mg/kg
B. Busulfan	4 mg/kg	q6h × 16 (days -7 to -4)	16 mg/kg
Cyclophosphamide	60 mg/kg	Daily × 2 (days -3, -2)	120 mg/kg

syngeneic (or autologous) marrow transplants, except in some cases of aplastic anemia that appear to be immune-mediated and may require immunosuppression with syngeneic marrow transplantation.

The degree of immunosuppression required for a successful allogeneic marrow transplant depends on several interrelated factors. These include the presence and severity of histoincompatibility, the extent of underlying immunosuppression resulting from the primary disease or its therapy, sensitization via previous exposure to allogeneic cells or tissues (especially via blood transfusions), and the number and type of marrow cells infused.

Histocompatibility

Experimentally, progressive degrees of histoincompatibility require more immunosuppression for sustained engraftment; human data are more limited but are consistent with this premise. For example, although current conditioning regimens that precede histocompatible marrow transplantation for leukemia are usually sufficiently immunosuppressive to prevent graft rejection, results in histoincompatible marrow transplantation indicate that they are not optimal. Aplastic anemia represents a somewhat different situation in that the additional immunosuppression offered by antineoplastic components such as TBI is not usually employed; consequently, graft rejection is a problem even in histocompatible recipients, chiefly in previously transfused patients who receive maximal doses (e.g., 200 mg/kg) of cyclophosphamide alone (see III.3). The use of a second immunosuppressive modality (e.g., antithymocyte globulin, total body or lymphoid irradiation) or donor buffy-coat transfusion reduces the risk of rejection in this situation.

Ideally, those patients whose transplants classically do not require immunosuppression (i.e., syngeneic and autologous sources) could avoid the use of such agents. However, due to the considerable overlap of function, as well as the need for multiple agents, this aspect is not usually exploited to a great degree.

Underlying Disease

In diseases with severe intrinsic immunodeficiency, and perhaps those in which concomitant immune defects are common (e.g., Hodgkin's disease), less immunosuppression is likely needed for allogeneic engraftment. This is usually not an important consideration, however, as the antineoplastic agents required to treat the underlying malignancy are severely immunosuppressive.

Sensitization

Blood transfusions given before transplantation sensitize patients against non-HLA histocompatibility determinants, and a previous history of blood transfusions is the chief prognostic factor in patients with severe aplastic anemia who reject HLA-identical transplants following cyclophosphamide alone. In patients with hematologic malignancies, however, additional antineoplastic therapy that is also immunosuppressive generally prevents graft rejection, at least in leukemic patients who receive unmanipulated HLA-identical marrow transplants. A history of prior transfusions from family members is rarely critical for leukemia patients (unlike aplastics); nevertheless, such should be avoided if possible.

Composition of the Graft

The composition of the marrow graft is undoubtedly an important determinant for the achievement of stable engraftment; unfortunately, it is currently still difficult to quantify the critical cells needed for stable engraftment (i.e., hematopoietic stem and accessory cells) due to a lack of suitable assays. Consequently, the "minimum engrafting dose" of hematopoietic stem cells in man is unknown – although total marrow nucleated cell doses of $<3 \times 10^8$/kg of body weight have been observed to be a negative prognostic sign for engraftment in certain aplastic anemia patients conditioned with cyclophosphamide before histocompatible marrow transplants. While it is likely that the minimum cell dose required for engraftment is less with syngeneic or autologous transplants, this observation is of limited clinical significance, since such amounts of marrow can usually be taken without difficulty (except for some cases of autologous harvests in extensively-pretreated patients).

The role of accessory cells in re-establishing stable hematopoiesis remains to be determined, although it has been observed that removing T-lymphocytes from the marrow to abrogate graft-versus-host disease (GVHD) (i.e., T-cell depletion) increases the risk of graft rejection, presumably because of a loss of an effect against surviving radioresistant host cells (see III.3). To overcome this effect, additional immunosuppression is required. However, this is a complicated proposition, as merely increasing the dose of chemotherapy drugs or irradiation may produce more immunosuppressive or antineoplastic effects but at the price of increased toxicity, and the use of other agents may be preferred; donor buffy-coat infusions post-transplantation, antithymocyte globulin, recombinant hematopoietic growth factors and certain monoclonal antibody complexes are examples.

Ablation of Unwanted Cell Populations

Although most marrow transplants have been performed for malignancies that involve the marrow (e.g., leukemias), there is no intrinsic reason that malignancies which do not involve the marrow (i.e., some malignant lymphomas and certain non-hematologic cancers) cannot be successfully treated with marrow transplantation regimens. In this circumstance, the transplant is primarily a "rescue" device after ablative-dose cytotoxic therapy, rather than performing both that function plus replacement of a diseased organ (although an immunologic antitumor function may be served in some cases of non-hematologic malignancy if allogeneic marrow is used). As noted above, the removal of a non-malignant cell population may also be necessary for some diseases and may require similar therapy as for a malignancy. There are even circumstances in which a qualitatively normal cell population must be ablated (e.g., in patients with aplastic anemia).

When malignant cells are present, the conditioning regimen is primarily aimed at their eradication, and the high recurrence rates that currently plague the use of marrow transplantation for malignancy underscore the inadequacy of current regimens. Over the past decade, the use of "early" transplantation (i.e., generally in first remission of acute leukemia or stable phase of chronic myelogenous leukemia) has been a more effective method of decreasing recurrence rates than has the use of more potent conditioning regimens. However, even with histocompatible marrow, recurrence rates of 20–40% have been observed; failures due to inadequate tumor ablation are especially common in non-hematologic malignant diseases.

One might think, therefore, that marrow transplantation should perhaps be limited to patients with early-stage disease. However, there are problems with this approach. Specifically, marrow transplant regimens are more toxic (and more expensive) than even intensive conventional therapy, which may be curative in some patients. Thus, especially for early-stage disease, marrow transplant regimens are indicated only when conventional regimens are unlikely to produce durable remissions. Moreover, it follows that as primary conventional therapy improves, it will become more difficult to justify marrow transplantation in early-stage disease – unless high-risk subgroups can be identified – and for some diseases, marrow transplant regimens may be more appropriately used as salvage therapy. Clearly, this is a complex situation that will change as both conventional and transplant-related therapies improve.

Major Conditioning Regimens in Current Use

The following sections briefly detail the rationale, the results, and general administration of several currently used regimens. It is not intended as a substitute for scrutiny of more complete reports, especially regarding details of dosing and administration. As noted above, a bewildering number of variations of several basic regimens have been used, and all methods of classification are artificial.

Chemoradiotherapy Regimens

Cyclophosphamide plus Total Body Irradiation

The pioneering efforts of Professor E.D. Thomas and his colleagues in the field of allogeneic marrow transplantation for hematologic malignancy have proved the efficacy of intensive chemoradiotherapy regimens, notably cyclophosphamide and TBI. In theory, TBI has unique benefits in the treatment of leukemia, such as the lack of cross-resistance to chemotherapeutic drugs, the ability to treat pharmacologic sanctuaries and the potent immunosuppression required for allogeneic marrow transplantation. Additional benefits of cyclophosphamide are assumed, as cyclophosphamide has been shown to possess both immunosuppressive and antitumor activity as a single agent in doses used in transplantation (e.g., 90–200 mg/kg). In any case, the non-hematologic toxicity spectrum of cyclophosphamide is different from TBI, and these agents do not obviously produce serious additive toxicity when used together.

A number of such regimens are currently in use (Table 9). The main differences involve the method of giving TBI, although varying cyclophosphamide doses (usually 120–200 mg/kg) have been employed. Cyclophosphamide doses of 120 mg/kg and fractionated TBI doses of ~1200 cGy (usually given as 200 cGy fractions, daily ×6 days or twice-daily ×3) are probably the most widely used, usually in the sequence of drug before radiotherapy (see Table 9,D). This regimen with cumulative TBI doses of 1575 cGy (usually given as 225 cGy daily ×7) is, as expected, more potent than a dose of 1200 cGy, but also more toxic, and is not as of yet routinely recommended.

As noted above, actuarial relapse rates following CY + TBI and histocompatible marrow transplantation in "early-stage" acute leukemia or chronic myelogenous leukemia are usually under 25%. However, when patients with advanced leukemia are transplanted, relapse rates rise to 50% or more. Therefore, while it may be argued that cyclophosphamide + TBI represents an adequate antileukemic regimen for early-stage leukemic patients, more effective methods will be required to increase cure rates in patients with leukemia advanced beyond initial remission or stable phase. The level of activity of cyclophosphamide + TBI is less clear with other hematologic malignancies, and it is unlikely that this regimen is suitable for most non-hematologic malignancies, as most solid tumors are not very responsive to high-dose cyclophosphamide and often are much less radiosensitive than hematologic cancers. With doses of TBI in excess of 1000 cGy, marrow ablation is usually assumed permanent, but in actuality is only variably so. The non-hematologic toxicity of cyclophosphamide + TBI is severe but largely reversible. Minor reversible complications include nausea, emesis, alopecia, mucositis, diarrhea, skin rash and abnormal liver function tests. More serious side effects include hemorrhagic cystitis, cardiomyopathy, veno-occlusive disease of the liver and interstitial pneumonitis. There are some data suggesting a chronic nephritis may be produced in some patients; other long-term effects include endocrine dysfunction and cataracts (see IV.4 and IV.5).

Cyclophosphamide plus Total Lymphoid Irradiation (TLI)

When radiotherapy is given primarily for its immunosuppressive rather than its antineoplastic effects, it is neither necessary nor desirable to irradiate the whole body, and toxicity to such radiosensitive organs as the lungs can be avoided to improve the therapeutic index of the conditioning by using TLI. TLI given in single doses of 300–750 cGy or fractionated doses in the range of 1200 cGy, has been substituted for TBI in patients with severe aplastic anemia at high risk for graft rejection following allogeneic marrow transplantation.

Cytarabine, With or Without Cyclophosphamide, Plus TBI (Table 10)

In leukemia patients, cytarabine has been used as conditioning in conventional dose (e.g., 100 mg/m^2 by continuous infusion daily × 5) with cyclophosphamide, in high dose (e.g., 3 gm/m^2 twice daily × 6) without cyclophosphamide, or in doses between these extremes with cyclophosphamide, before TBI. Conventional-dose cytarabine plus cyclophosphamide (120 mg/kg) and single-fraction TBI (500 cGy) at a high dose rate has been found useful in chronic myelogenous leukemia in an initial stable phase, while the high-dose (i.e., 3 gm/m^2) regimen (without cyclophosphamide) has been used in acute lymphoblastic leukemia in second remission with fractionated TBI (1200 cGy).

Etoposide, With or Without Cyclophosphamide, Plus TBI (Table 10)

Etoposide (i.e., 60 mg/kg × 1) has been used after 1320 cGy hyperfractionated TBI in high-risk acute leukemia with encouraging preliminary results. Although this regimen is of interest, it should not be used without cyclophosphamide in situations in which additional immunosuppression is required (e.g., T-cell depletion or histoincompatibility). These three agents have also been used by other investigators, arguably with increased toxicity.

Comparison of These Regimens

Comparative studies have involved the TBI dose several. The TBI dose of 1200 cGy (again, usually given as 200 cGy twice-daily × 3 or daily × 6) is as effective as, if not better than, other doses in producing durable remission; higher TBI doses produce better antileukemic effects but at the cost of greater toxicity. More recently, a comparative study has indicated better results with a cyclophosphamide and TBI regimen than with a busulfan and cyclophosphamide regimen.

Moreover, there may be cases in which a regimen is preferred due to an anticipation of better antineoplastic effects (e.g., etoposide rather than cyclophosphamide) or toxicity (e.g., prior hemorrhagic cystitis with cyclophosphamide). Although such choices seem reasonable, they are of unproven benefit.

Chemotherapy Regimens

Cyclophosphamide

Generally speaking, cyclophosphamide doses should be calculated on the basis of ideal body weight or body surface area calculated using ideal body weight. Other considerations regarding the use of cyclophosphamide in any regimen include the avoidance of patients with serious preexisting cardiac disease if possible, and those with abnormal urinary function, especially if due to obstructive uropathy. The former is discussed below; the latter is important since good renal and urologic function is required to excrete the toxic metabolite acrolein, which produces excessive uroepithelial damage unless diluted and excreted promptly.

Accordingly, suitable hydration is vital to minimize severe hemorrhagic cystitis; cyclophosphamide has an antidiuretic hormone (ADH)-like effect on the kidney that complicates this requirement. One method of hyperhydration utilizes a cystalloid intravenous solution at $\geqslant 3 \, L/m^2/day$, initiated before cyclophosphamide is given to establish good urine flow, and continued for 48 hours after the last dose. Prophylactic diuretics (e.g., furosemide 10–20 mg iv) are given immediately after cyclophosphamide, and as needed to keep a urine output of $\geqslant 100$ ml per hour. Additional diuretic is used to keep the morning body weight within 1–2 kg of baseline. Alternatively, the uroprotectant 2-mercaptoethane sulphonate (mesna) can be used with less hyperhydration – but without clear-cut additional benefit except in circumstances in which the volume of fluid infused is a major consideration. Bladder irrigation is of no obvious additional benefit.

A severe hemorrhagic myopericarditis is occasionally seen with high-dose cyclophosphamide; it is highly lethal and is usually observed with doses in the range of (and especially in excess of) 200 mg/kg. Due to the devastating consequences of this rare complication, it is reasonable to assume that cardiac compromise of any etiology may predispose its occurrence. However, this assumption is unproven, as cardiomyopathy certainly occurs in patients without a prior history of cardiac disease.

In untransfused patients with aplastic anemia, intravenous cyclophosphamide 50 mg/kg daily × 4 (total dose = 200 mg/kg) produces stable engraftment with a low rate of rejection. This is usually the only situation in which cyclophosphamide is employed as a single agent.

Busulfan Plus Cyclophosphamide (Table 11)

This regimen was developed by Professor G.W. Santos and colleagues to avoid the use of TBI, and substitutes busulfan 1 mg/kg given orally every 6 hours × 16 doses (total dose 16 mg/kg of ideal body weight) combined with cyclophosphamide 50 mg/kg IV daily × 4 (= 200 mg/kg). Tutschka, et al have used the same busulfan dose with a lower dose of cyclophosphamide (i.e., 60 mg/kg × 2), and reported less toxicity. (However, the variability in the pharmacokinetics of busulfan and the relationship of higher "areas under the curves" and hepatic toxicity cast some doubt on this postulate, at least concerning the liver. Moreover, dose-adjusted busulfan therapy will likely become routine within the near future.) Lower doses of busulfan (i.e., 8–12 mg/kg) with cyclophosphamide (200 mg/kg) have been used in conditioning regimens for non-malignant disease (e.g., thalassemia major).

In contrast to cyclophosphamide plus TBI (discussed below), immediate side effects – specifically nausea and emesis, skin changes and mucositis – are less. However, patients may vomit doses of busulfan, thereby complicating dosing, and routine antiemetics should be considered. Also, it should be emphasized that different busulfan pharmacokinetics apply to small children. The serious toxicity of busulfan plus cyclophosphamide tends to be hepatic veno-occlusive disease; there is also a suggestion of an increased rate of hemorrhagic cystitis with this regimen versus cyclophosphamide plus TBI. Generalized seizures also have been observed in some cases, especially when adequate levels of prophylactic phenytoin have not been given.

A direct comparison of the conditioning regimens of busulfan plus cyclophosphamide and cyclophosphamide plus TBI has been reported for acute myelogenous leukemia in an initial remission, and it appears the chemoradiotherapy regimen is better, although dose-adjustment of busulfan may produce improved results. The main reason for selecting busulfan plus cyclophosphamide over a TBI regimen would be the avoidance of patients with prior mediastinal radiotherapy – a known risk factor for idiopathic interstitial pneumonitis. Both regimens produce similar growth rate impairment in children.

A number of variants of busulfan plus cyclophosphamide have been tested, adding (or substituting) cytarabine, etoposide, melphalan and even TBI. Again, preliminary results are interesting, but no definite recommendation can be made at this time regarding these modifications.

BACT Variants

Also in an attempt to avoid the toxicity of TBI, the BACT regimen (carmustine [BCNU], cytarabine [ara-C], cyclophosphamide and thioguanine) was developed at the National Cancer Institute (U.S.) in the 1970s. As discussed above, it is somewhat unusual in that only cyclophosphamide is used in near-maximal doses. Subsequently, this regimen was found to be ineffective in advanced acute leukemia, but has utility in the treatment of certain lymphomas (notably Burkitt's lymphoma).

BACT has been extensively modified and is currently used only rarely in its original form, usually in Burkitt's lymphoma patients. Major modifications include CBV (cyclophosphamide, BCNU [carmustine] and etoposide [VP16-213]), BEAM (BCNU, etoposide, cytarabine and melphalan) and BAVC (BCNU, cytarabine, VP16-213 and cyclophosphamide), regimens used to treat various hematologic cancers, primarily (but not exclusively) with autologous marrow transplants. In some of these regimens, most or all agents are escalated to near-maximal doses.

Other modifications have been developed and are undergoing clinical use. This is especially the case for breast cancer, for which cyclophosphamide, carmustine, melphalan, thioTEPA and carboplatin have been used in various combinations and schedules.

Related Approaches

Pre-Conditioning Cytoreduction

The importance of the conventional therapy used to produce initial cytoreduction before conditioning and transplantation should not be underestimated. For a variety of reasons, transplantation has only rarely been employed as primary therapy for neoplastic disease, usually in circumstances in which normal primary therapy is ineffective in producing initial remissions (such as myelodysplasia), and most workers prefer to use marrow transplant regimens to "consolidate" a complete remission as produced by conventional therapy. Therefore, the effectiveness of primary conventional therapy may be of critical importance, as the "depth" of remission is presumably a major factor in determining the subsequent success of the conditioning regimens. Both this factor, as well as the cumulative toxic effects of these agents may be difficult to quantitate, but certainly are important determinants of post-transplant toxicity.

Despite the pivotal role of initial conventional cytoreduction to produce remission in some diseases, observations to date do not clearly support the use of additional conventional chemotherapy to further treat the underlying disease before transplantation. For instance, acute leukemia patients in complete remission generally do not require extensive consolidation chemotherapy prior to elective allogeneic transplantation unless a lengthy delay is anticipated. Even in patients with relapsed hematologic malignancy the desirability of conventional cytoreduction is uncertain – although it has become common practice to use conventional therapy as "chemosensitivity testing" in the non-Hodgkin's lymphomas.

Therefore, although controversial and difficult to generalize, a previously-treated patient in whom marrow transplantation is indicated should generally be transplanted promptly, as the use of additional conventional chemotherapy may or may not significantly enhance cell kill but is likely to produce cumulative toxicity predisposing the patient to complications that may compromise or obviate transplantation. There are undoubtedly many exceptions to this postulate; in some cases, chemotherapy may be needed merely to control the underlying disease process until a transplant can be arranged.

There are also circumstances in which special methods of cytoreduction are indicated; for example, bulk tumor deposits in the central nervous system, gonads or lymph nodes may be treated with additional local radiotherapy. (As above, conventional involved-field radiotherapy to the mediastinum should be avoided if a conditioning regimen including TBI is planned, as such therapy predisposes to fatal interstitial pneumonitis.) Intrathecal chemotherapy to control meningeal leukemia may also be required.

Post-Transplantation Therapy

In some respects, therapy given after transplantation is attractive, as minimal tumor burden may exist especially in patients not at high risk of a recurrence. However, conventional chemotherapeutic or radiotherapeutic methods employed post-transplant are excessively toxic, since the status of the transplanted marrow (and the patient as well!) is fragile in the early post-grafting period.

Less myelosuppressive therapies are more attractive. For instance, manipulation of the "graft-versus-leukemia" effect (see III and IV) as a post-transplant modality has some attractive features. Since mortality is more common in acute than in chronic GVHD, perhaps the latter could be provoked in a mild form that would be actively antileukemic without being excessively toxic. In any case, however, the ability to precisely modulate either of these processes is currently very limited. Of course, it may be possible to avoid GVHD but exploit a similar antineoplastic effect, as detailed in III.2. Related measures such as α-interferon, various immunotoxins and cytokines (e.g., IL-2) are now being evaluated in this regard.

Radioimmunopharmaceuticals

Although radioimmunopharmaceuticals are investigational as of this writing, they appear to hold promise in the development of improved conditioning regimens. Specifically, the demonstrated dose effect of radiotherapy, the intrinsic radiosensitivity of most hematologic malignancies, and the potential selectivity of monoclonal antibodies make this an area of immense potential interest.

Conditioning for Second Transplants

In general, second transplants are considered in two circumstances: graft rejection in patients with aplastic anemia, and systemic recurrence of hematologic malignancy. While both situations are desperate, the latter is usually more so, since conditioning for aplastic anemia rarely produces cumulative toxicity to the extent that a second course of conditioning cannot be given, and the addition of another immunosuppressive agent (e.g., TBI or antithymocyte globulin [ATG]) may be useful. The problem with recurrent leukemia is different. Presumably, a potent antileukemic regimen was used initially and the second regimen must eradicate a more refractory leukemia to be successful. Furthermore, since many patients will have been exposed to near tissue-tolerance levels of cytotoxics, cumulative toxicity (especially to the liver or lung) may be present, precluding safe administration of a conditioning regimen. However, there are usually other considerations, and highly selected patients with hematologic malignancy, especially those with a remission after the first marrow transplant lasting >1 year, may be considered for second transplants. In the usual case, patients who received TBI initially should get a chemotherapy regimen with the second transplant, and vice versa; nevertheless, a high incidence of severe regimen-related toxicity should be anticipated.

Approaches to Improving Conditioning Regimens

Unless a formal clinical research study is planned, it is prudent to use an established conditioning regimen rather than to construct a novel regimen. Likewise, if modifications of an existing conditioning regimen are deemed essential in a particular case, minimal deviations from the standard regimen are recommended.

The need to develop new conditioning regimens, especially for the hematologic malignancies, depends in some respects upon one's view of the role of marrow transplantation in these diseases. For example, if marrow transplantation for acute leukemia (from histocompatible related donors) is only used to consolidate the first remission state, it will be very difficult to prove the efficacy of justify a more intensive conditioning regimen. On the other hand, if marrow transplant regimens are used mainly in patients who fail primary chemotherapy, then alternative tactics including intensification of current conditioning regimens may become important.

In any case, several factors deserve consideration in the construction of a new conditioning regimen:

1. The goal in constructing a new regimen is to improve survival, and a correlation exists between dose-intensity, antineoplastic effects and toxicity. This is exemplified by the Seattle experience with cyclophosphamide 120 mg/kg plus the 1575 cGy (225 cGy daily × 7) dose of TBI versus the more usual 1200 cGy (200 cGy daily × 6) dose. In this experience, the higher dose was a more effective in an antileukemic sense, but did not improve survival due to a greater degree of toxicity. Moreover, these toxicities are likely complex; for instance, the TBI 1575 cGy regimen produces more mucosal toxicity and may prevent the use of full doses of methotrexate and thus increase GVHD. Therefore, mere augmentation of doses of current components may or may not be very useful.

    Conversely, the above data should not be used to conclude that more effective regimens are always too toxic, as better knowledge of pharmacokinetics as well as the availability of new agents (e.g., radioimmunopharmaceuticals) and perhaps of selective cytoprotective agents will evolve and be useful. The point to be emphasized is that a systematic approach to this problem is necessary, and innovative methods of improving the therapeutic index will likely be required. Obviously, the difficulty in the development of improved and especially novel regimens should not be underestimated.

2. If the regimen is to be used for allogeneic marrow transplantation, potent immunosuppression is required. As

noted earlier, while this is neither necessary nor desirable for syngeneic or autologous bone marrow transplantation regimens, it is difficult to avoid. Also, a more potent immunosuppressive regimen may be needed for durable engraftment in certain situations (e.g., T-cell depletion in histoincompatible transplants), and novel methods of producing same (i.e., not merely by augmenting the dose of current regimens or adding more existing agents) should be considered.

3. While it will be difficult to develop unique conditioning regimens for each disease, especially malignancies, it is also difficult to believe that one or two regimens will be optimal for all diseases; nevertheless, few workers believe a wide range of conditioning regimens is needed – or is even possible to develop. As a general rule, conditioning used for antineoplastic effects should contain elements that have some degree of activity in conventional dose but were not used in the primary therapy, both to avoid cumulative toxicity and especially to minimize the exposure of resistant cells to previously used agents. As previously noted with BACT, it is not necessary that all agents in a conditioning regimen be used in augmented doses. The use of some agents in conventional dose might be considered in certain patients when a particularly desirable agent is not suitable for dose escalation but was not extensively used in primary therapy; examples include cisplatin or anthracyclines.

4. The superiority of a new versus a standard regimen may be difficult to prove. For instance, as noted above, determining the relative effectiveness of standard versus test regimens in acute myelogenous leukemia during first remission will require a large randomized trial. Moreover, especially when transplantation is delayed until end-stage malignancy is present, such patients are often heavily pretreated and have resultant organ dysfunction (clinical or subclinical) that may increase post-transplant toxicity. This is a difficult problem, especially with the relatively uncommon hematologic malignancies, and one that should be fully considered when Phase I-II studies are planned.

Future Developments in Conditioning Regimens

Within the past few years, there has been a growing cynicism that either the optimization of existing regimens or the construction of new regimens will markedly improve cure rates. Nevertheless, the situation of a "zero-sum equation" (i.e., more therapy produces more antineoplastic activity but also produces more fatal toxicity) is likely not absolute, and further clinical trials are indicated. Conversely, although new agents – either existing but previously-unused cytotoxic drugs or perhaps truly unique agents – might produce improved conditioning regimens, this will not necessarily be the case and may not be possible unless novel cytoprotective strategies are developed. In the absence of strikingly improved new regimens, the goal of better results may be attained, to a degree, by providing optimal, standardized initial therapy to all suitable patients and by performing marrow transplantation at the earliest appropriate moment.

References

Atkinson K, Biggs J, Noble G, Ashby M, Concannon A, Dodds A (1987) Preparative regimens for marrow transplantation containing busulphan are associated with haemorrhagic cystitis and hepatic veno-occlusive disease but a short duration of leucopenia and little oro-pharyngeal mucositis. Bone Marrow Transplant 2:385

Aurer I, Gale RP (1991) Are new conditioning regimens for transplants in acute myelogenous leukemia better? Bone Marrow Transplant 7:255

Blaise D, Maraninchi D, Archimbaud E, Reiffers J, Devergie A, Jouet JP, Milpied N, Attal M, Michallet M, Ifrah N, Kuentz M, Dauriac C, Bordigoni P, Gratecos N, Guilhot F, Guyotat D, Gouvernet J, Gluckman E (1992) Allogeneic bone marrow transplantation for acute myeloid leukemia in first remission: A randomized trial of busulfan-cytoxan versus cytoxan-total body irradiation as preparative regimen: A report from the Groupe d'Etudes de la Greffe de Moelle Osseuse. Blood 79:2578

Blume KG, Forman SJ, O'Donnell MR, Doroshow JH, Krance RA, Nademanee AP, Snyder DS, Schmidt GM, Fahey JL, Metter GE, Hill LR, Findley DO, Sniecinski IJ (1987) Total body irradiation and high-dose etoposide: A new preparatory regimen for bone marrow transplantation in patients with advanced hematologic malignancies. Blood 69:1015

Clift RA, Buckner CD, Appelbaum FR, Bearman SI, Petersen FB, Fisher LD, Anasetti C, Beatty P, Bensinger WI, Doney K, Hill RS, McDonald

GB, Martin P, Sanders J, Singer J, Stewart P, Sullivan KM, Witherspoon R, Storb R, Hansen JA, Thomas ED (1990) Allogeneic marrow transplantation in patients with acute myeloid leukemia in first remission: A randomized trial of two irradiation regimens. Blood 76:1867

Clift RA, Buckner CD, Appelbaum FR, Bryant E, Bearman SI, Petersen FB, Fisher LD, Anasetti C, Beatty P, Bensinger WI, Doney K, Hill RS, McDonald GB, Martin P, Meyers J, Sanders J, Singer J, Stewart P, Sullivan KM, Witherspoon R, Storb R, Hansen JA, Thomas ED (1991) Allogeneic marrow transplantation in patients with chronic myeloid leukemia in the chronic phase: A randomized trial of two irradiation regimens. Blood 77:1660

Coccia PF, Strandjord SE, Warkentin PI, Cheung N-V, Gordon EM, Novak LJ, Shina DC, Herzig RH (1988) High-dose cytosine arabinoside and fractionated total-body irradiation: An improved preparative regimen for bone marrow transplantation of children with acute lymphoblastic leukemia in remission. Blood 71:888

Fischer A, Friedrich W, Fasth A, Blanche S, Le Deist F, Girault D, Veber F, Vossen J, Lopez M, Griscelli C, Hirn M (1991) Reduction of graft failure by a monoclonal antibody (anti-LFA-1 CD11a) after HLA non-identical bone marrow transplantation in children with immunodeficiencies, osteopetrosis, and Fanconi's anemia: A European Group for Immunodeficiency/European Group for BMT Report. Blood 77: 249

Fischer A, Griscelli C, Blanche S, Le Deist F, Veber F, Lopez M, Delaage M, Olive D, Mawas C, Mawas C, Janossy G (1986) Prevention of graft failure by an anti-HLFA-1 monoclonal antibody in HLA-mismatched bone-marrow transplantation. Lancet 2:1058

Graw Jr RG, Lohrmann H-P, Bull MI, Decter J, Herzig GP, Bull JM, Leventhal BG, Yankee RA, Herzig RH, Krueger GRF, Bleyer WA, Buja ML, McGinniss MH, Alter HJ, Whang-Peng J, Gralnick HR, Kirkpatrick CH, Henderson ES (1974) Bone-marrow transplantation following combination chemotherapy immunosuppression (B.A.C.T.) in patients with acute leukemia. Transplant Proc 6:349

Gribben JG, Linch DC, Singer CRJ, McMillan AK, Jarrett M, Goldstone AH (1989) Successful treatment of refractory Hodgkin's disease by high-dose combination chemotherapy and autologous bone marrow transplantation. Blood 73:340

Grochow LB, Jones RJ, Brundrett RB, Braine HG, Chen T-L, Saral R, Santos GW, Colvin OM (1989) Pharmacokinetics of busulfan: Correlation with veno-occlusive disease in patients undergoing bone marrow transplantation. Cancer Chemother Pharmacol 25:55

Grochow LB, Krivit W, Whitley CB, Blazar B (1990) Busulfan disposition in children. Blood 75:1723

Grossbard ML, Freedman AS, Ritz J, Coral F, Goldmacher VS, Eliseo L, Spector N, Dear K, Lambert JM, Blattler WA, Taylor JA, Nadler LM (1992) Serotherapy of B-cell neoplasms with anti-B4-blocked ricin: A phase I trial of daily bolus infusion. Blood 79:576

Herzig GP, Herzig RH (1990) Current concepts in dose intensity and marrow transplantation. Acute Myelogenous Leukemia: Progress and Controversies, Gale RP (ed), Wiley-Liss, New York:333

Jagannath S, Dicke KA, Armitage JO, Cabanillas FF, Horwitz LJ, Vellekoop L, Zander AR, Spitzer G (1986) High-dose cyclophosphamide, carmustine, and etoposide and autologous bone marrow transplantation for relapsed Hodgkin's disease. Ann Intern Med 104: 163

Klingemann H-G, Grigg AP, Wilkie-Boyd K, Barnett MJ, Eaves AC, Reece DE, Shepherd JD, Phillips GL (1991) Treatment with recombinant interferon (α-2β) early after bone marrow transplantation in patients at high risk for relapse. Blood 78:3306

Lucarelli G, Galimberti M, Polchi P, Angelucci E, Baronciani D, Giardini C, Politi P, Durazzi SMT, Muretto P, Albertini F (1990) Bone marrow transplantation in patients with thalassemia. N Engl J Med 322:417

Parkman R, Rappeport JM, Hellman S, Lipton J, Smith B, Geha R, Nathan DG (1984) Busulfan and total body irradiation as antihematopoietic stem cell agents in the preparation of patients with congenital bone marrow disorders for allogeneic bone marrow transplantation. Blood 64:852

Pecego R, Hill R, Appelbaum FR, Amos D, Buckner CD, Fefer A, Thomas ED (1986) Interstitial pneumonitis following autologous bone marrow transplantation. Transplantation 42:515

Ramsay NKC, Kim TH, McGlave P (1983) Total lymphoid irradiation and cyclophosphamide conditioning prior to bone marrow transplantation for patients with severe aplastic anemia. Blood 62:622

Reece DE, Barnett MJ, Connors JM, Fairey RN, Fay JW, Greer JP, Herzig GP, Herzig RH, Klingemann H-G, LeMaistre CF, O'Reilly SE, Shepherd JD, Spinelli JJ, Voss NJ, Wolff SN, Phillips GL (1991) Intensive chemotherapy with cyclophosphamide, carmustine, and etoposide followed by autologous bone marrow transplantation for relapsed Hodgkin's disease. J Clin Oncol 9:1871

Santos GW, Tutschka PJ, Brookmeyer R, Saral R, Beschorner WE, Bias WB, Braine HG, Burns WH, Elfenbein GJ, Kaizer H, Mellits D, Sensenbrenner LL, Stuart RK, Yeager AM (1983) Marrow transplantation for acute nonlymphocytic leukemia after treatment with busulfan and cyclophosphamide. N Engl J Med 309:1347

Slavin S (1987) Total lymphoid irradiation. Immunol Today 8:88

Soiffer RJ, Murray C, Cochran K, Cameron C, Wang E, Schow PW, Daley JF, Ritz J (1992) Clinical and immunologic effects of prolonged infusion of low-dose recombinant interleukin-2 after autologous and T-cell-depleted allogeneic bone marrow transplantation. Blood 79:517

Storb R, Doney KC, Thomas ED (1982) Marrow transplantation with or without donor buffy coat cells for 65 transfused aplastic anemia patients. Blood 59:236

Storb R, Thomas ED, Buckner CD (1980) Marrow transplantation in thirty "untransfused" patients with severe aplastic anemia. Ann Intern Med 92:30

Tutschka PJ, Copelan EA, Klein JP (1987) Bone marrow transplantation for leukemia following a new busulfan and cyclophosphamide regimen. Blood 70:1382

van Bekkum DW (1984) Conditioning regimens for marrow grafting. Semin Hematol 21:81

Wheeler C, Antin JH, Churchill WH, Come SE, Smith BR, Bubley GJ, Rosenthal DS, Rappaport JM, Ault KA, Schnipper LE, Eder JP (1990) Cyclophosphamide, carmustine, and etoposide with autologous bone marrow transplantation in refractory Hodgkin's disease and non-Hodgkin's lymphoma: A dose-finding study. J Clin Oncol 8:648

2. Collection, Processing and Infusion of Marrow

Overview

One of the functions of the preparative or conditioning regimen before marrow infusion is to create space for the transplanted autologous or allogeneic donor marrow. Marrow for transplantation can be obtained from a healthy related or unrelated donor, or in some cases the patient's own "autologous" marrow may be used. In both situations, the marrow is harvested, and certain manipulations may be performed, before infusion into the patient after the conditioning regimen has been completed. Intravenously-infused donor or autologous marrow cells reseed in the marrow cavity of the recipient, a process known as "homing", and start to replicate and differentiate.

In the discussion that follows, the term "donor" refers to both allogeneic and autologous marrow donors, except where otherwise noted.

Marrow Harvest

Harvest Procedure

Bone marrow harvesting is performed under sterile conditions in the operating room, usually by two members of the Transplant Team. The procedure requires about 1–2 hours with the donor under general anesthesia. In donors with contraindications for general anesthesia, or if preferred by the donor, epidural anesthesia can be performed instead. The site of marrow aspiration is usually the posterior iliac crests; if a high nucleated cell count is required, the anterior iliac crests are harvested as well. The practice of using just the posterior pelvis has the advantage of shortening the anesthesia and procedure time by eliminating the need to turn the donor. Occasionally, in situations where a large marrow dose is desired, such as in patients with aplastic anemia or when there is a major size disparity between a smaller donor and a larger recipient, marrow is also taken from the sternum. In children who serve as donors for adult patients, the upper third of the tibiae may also be used for aspiration. On average, $2-10 \times 10^8$ mononuclear cells/kg recipient weight are harvested for an allogeneic marrow graft, and about $1-3 \times 10^8$ cells/kg for an autologous marrow graft. Increased donor age is associated with a slight reduction in the number of nucleated cells collected per ml of marrow, and therefore a larger volume may be required from older donors. If the donor is <10 years of age a median cell number of 4.5×10^8/kg donor weight can be expected. This figure drops to 2.8×10^8/kg in the 10–20 years age group. Donors between the age of 20 and 60 years have a median yield of 2.2×10^8/kg whereas this number drops to 2.0×10^8/kg in the donors older than 60 years.

The needles used for marrow harvesting are 6–10 cm long with a ball or knob handle (Fig. 1). Prior to the procedure, the aspiration syringes are rinsed with a solution consisting of tissue culture medium mixed with heparin. Through puncture sites in the skin, about 5–10 aspirations are performed with the needle point being moved vertically a few millimeters for each aspiration. While the needle is rotated to expose the bevel to different areas of marrow space, vigorous suction is applied. The marrow is then expelled into a beaker or collection bag containing heparinized tissue culture medium.

About 150–300 aspirations are required to obtain the required number of nucleated cells. Some peripheral blood will be included in the aspirate; it is not advisable to take

Fig. 1. a Marrow aspiration equipment including needles and glass syringes (*1*), stand with beakers (*2*) and screen (*3*). **b** With a different collection system, bone marrow is collected into a bag containing an anticoagulant. It is then filtered through several progressively finer mesh filters into a second bag and infused into the patient. (Photograph supplied courtesy of the Fenwal Division of Baxter Healthcare Corporation)

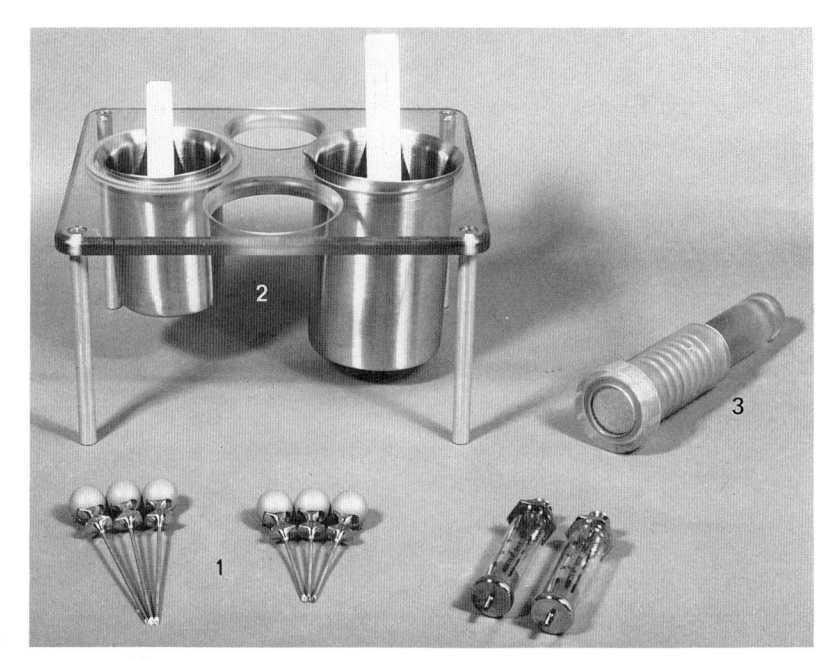

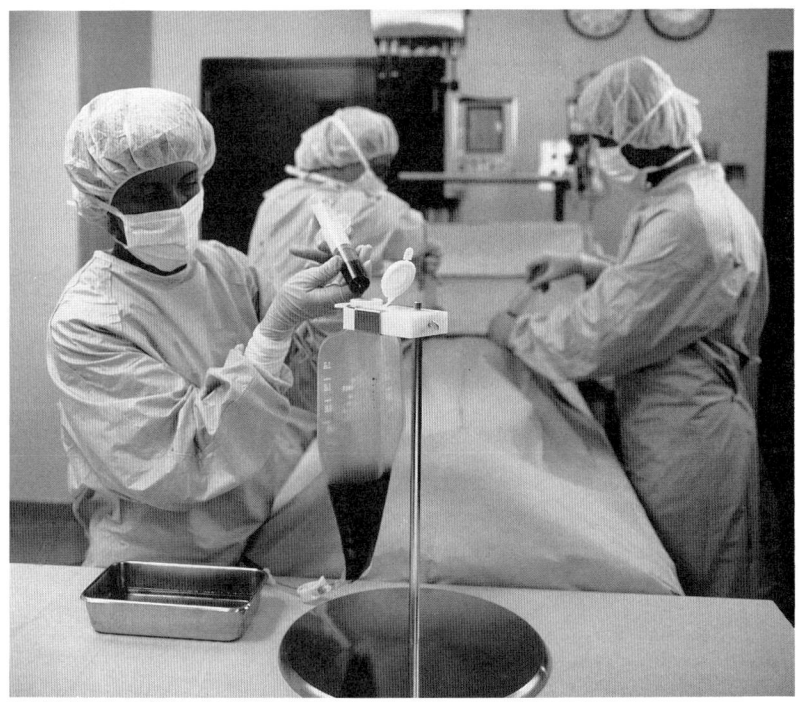

Collection, Processing and Infusion of Marrow 91

more than 3–5 ml of marrow with a single aspiration, as this may cause an increase in the amount of peripheral blood containing T-lymphocytes that is included. This is undesirable at least with allogeneic transplantation because of the increased risk of GVHD.

After marrow aspiration is completed, the marrow is passed through coarse and fine mesh filters into a second beaker or bag collection system (Fig. 1). This filtration step is required to remove bone or fat particles and tissue fragments and to break up cell aggregates that might cause pulmonary emboli in the recipient. After marrow samples have been taken for culture and cell counting, the marrow is placed into a standard blood transfer pack for immediate intravenous infusion into the patient or for further processing and/or storage where appropriate.

Risks Involved in Marrow Harvest

The risks for the marrow donor are primarily confined to those of anesthesia. An analysis of over 3000 harvest procedures showed that virtually all donors experienced pain at the marrow aspiration site for a few days following the harvest. Only 9 donors (0.3%) had potentially life-threatening complications, infectious or cardiovascular in nature, and all recovered uneventfully. However, there is an unpublished observation of one donor who could not be resuscitated following a cardiac arrest during anesthesia. Other donors have experienced a transient cardio-respiratory arrest but have been resuscitated successfully. Spinal anesthesia can cause post-spinal headache and occasionally urinary retention. Infections or prolonged bleeding from the marrow harvest site occur rarely, and the hospitalization time for the allogeneic donor is usually 1–2 days. Some centers perform marrow harvests in an out-patient setting; the donor is harvested early in the morning and sent home in the evening. Usually the allogeneic donor does not require any blood support perioperatively, although most centers prefer to collect and store a unit of the donor's own "autologous" blood about 1 week before the harvest, for transfusion during or after marrow harvest if necessary. This avoids the risk of acquiring a transfusion-related disease, as may occur with allogeneic transfusion.

The situation is different for patients undergoing an autologous marrow harvest. These patients usually have already been exposed to blood products (e.g., during induction chemotherapy) and likely will receive additional transfusions during the transplant course as well. These patients, therefore, do not need an autologous blood unit taken before marrow harvest.

Marrow Storage

Allogeneic Marrow

Allogeneic marrow may remain untreated or be transferred to the laboratory for marrow processing (see below). If the harvested marrow is not to be processed further, it will be immediately transferred from the operating room to the transplantation ward and prepared for infusion into the patient. However, if immediate infusion is not possible (e.g., when donor and patient are located in different cities), the marrow can be kept viable at 4°C for some time. It is not known exactly how long human marrow can be kept viable, but successful engraftment has been obtained with marrow stored at 4°C for up to 48 hours after harvesting. Allogeneic marrow can also be frozen or "cryopreserved"; this has been done infrequently but should be considered in circumstances in which timing of the marrow harvest relative to the transplant may be a problem. The storage of allogeneic marrow may become more popular as it could facilitate the logistics of marrow donation, especially for unrelated donors.

Autologous Marrow

In the autologous transplant situation, some diseases (e.g., malignant lymphomas and solid tumors) may not involve the bone marrow, and this "clean" autologous marrow can then be harvested and stored without further processing to be re-infused at a later date. In other diseases involving the bone marrow, in particular acute leukemia, autologous marrow can only be used once a marrow remission has been induced. For example, a patient with acute myeloid leukemia may have marrow harvested in first remission, frozen and stored for use at the time of subsequent relapse or after achieving a second remission. However, some investigators feel strongly that even marrow that is morphologically in remission should be submitted to a cleaning or purging procedure before infusion or cryopreservation (see below).

Cryopreservation

Autologous bone marrow is generally stored using dimethylsulfoxide (DMSO) as a cryopreservant. A buffy coat containing the nucleated cells is removed from the marrow by centrifugation in a standard blood-transfer pack using devices such as the IBM 2991 Blood Cell Processor, Sorvall RC-3B centrifuge or the CS 3000 blood cell separator. The buffy coat is resuspended in medium mixed with 10% DMSO and placed in plastic bags, usually at between 75–150 ml/bag. Numerous brands of freezing bags, often made of Kapton/Teflon film, are available. These bags are frozen in a controlled rate freezer at $-1°C$ per minute to a temperature of $-60°C$ then at $-5°C$ per minute to a temperature of $-90°C$, and then transferred to the liquid phase of a liquid-nitrogen freezer. Contamination during *in vitro* processing is rare and does not constitute an increased risk for the patient. Some loss in viability and cell number can occur during the freezing and thawing procedure; therefore, cell viability before and after freezing must be determined ideally by colony forming unit assay. Recovery of hemopoietic progenitor cell (or "stem cell") function after freezing and thawing should be on the order of 90% of that obtained with fresh cells. In addition, microbiological cultures should be taken before freezing and after thawing, to exclude bacterial and fungal contamination of the stored marrow.

Frozen marrow can be used successfully for marrow transplants after many years of storage; however, transplant centers have different policies in terms of how long they will store a patient's marrow.

Manipulation of Bone Marrow

Several modalities for *in vitro* treatment of the harvested marrow have been developed aimed at removing either red blood cells or T-lymphocytes from allogeneic marrow, (red blood cell or T-cell depletion) or malignant cells from autologous marrow (tumor cell purging).

Red Blood Cell and Plasma Depletion

In case of ABO incompatibility between recipient and donor (e.g., recipient: O, donor: B), red blood cells and mononuclear cells can be separated either by conventional density gradient techniques (such as Percoll) or more frequently by the use of special centrifuges or cell washers.

If the recipient has a high antibody titer against the donor's blood type (major ABO mismatch), some centers perform several sessions of plasmapheresis until the titers is significantly lowered; this procedure is considered necessary in situations in which red cells cannot be (or have not been) reliably removed from the donor marrow or if the recipient's antibody titer are high, as there is some concern that blood group antigens are also expressed on hematopoietic precursor cells. Conversely, if the donor has an antibody, usually an isoagglutinine, against the recipient's blood type, the plasma must be separated from the donor marrow before infusion.

Blood transfusion after transplantation should be of the recipient's ABO type until engraftment. Thereafter cells carrying donor type antigens should be transfused. B-lymphocytes of the recipient may survive for some time (3–4 months) after transplantation and may produce antibodies, which can cause hemolytic anemia with increased transfusion requirements in cases with major patient/donor ABO incompatibilities.

T-Lymphocyte Depletion (Table 12; see also III.2.)

T-lymphocytes in allogeneic donor marrow can initiate acute GVHD in the recipient; removing them before marrow infusion decreases the incidence of GVHD. Most commonly,

Table 12. Methods of in vitro T-cell depletion

Monoclonal antibodies and complement
Monoclonal antibodies coupled to
– Magnetic beads
– Immunotoxins
Lectin (soybean) agglutination
Counterflow centrifugal elutriation
Chemoseparation

T-cell depletion is accomplished by the use of monoclonal antibodies against T-cells with or without the use of complement (cytolytic treatment). Immunotoxins such as ricin chain A conjugated to monoclonal antibodies may also be used instead of complement. Donor T-cells can also be removed by lectin and sheep red blood cell agglutination or by the use of magnetic beads coated with monoclonal antibodies against T-cell surface antigens. In addition, mechanical methods such as counterflow elutriation are being employed (see III.2). Unfortunately, complete removal of donor-T-lymphocytes has increased the risk of graft failure as well as the risk of relapse of the underlying malignancy. This has led to the development of protocols aimed at depleting only certain T-cell fractions (selective T-cell depletion) or to return cytotoxic killer cells to the marrow before infusion.

Tumor Cell Purging

When autologous marrow is used for transplantation, clonogenic leukemia, lymphoma or other malignant cells potentially present at the time of marrow harvest could lead to disease recurrence. Therefore, pharmacological, immunological or physical techniques are employed in an attempt to remove or "purge" residual tumor cells.

For in vitro purging, generally a buffy coat of nucleated cells is prepared from the harvested marrow. This cell suspension is then mixed (e.g., at 37°C for 30 minutes) with autologous plasma and tissue culture medium along with a cytotoxic drug (such as 4-hydroperoxycyclophosphamide or mafosfamide, derivatives of cyclophosphamide aimed at destroying malignant cells) or a monoclonal antibody directed at malignant B-cell or T-cell markers or other reagents. In the case of monoclonal antibody treatment, a second or third incubation with complement is often needed to lyse the target cells, followed by several washing steps, before the marrow can be frozen or reinfused into the recipient. Purging procedures must be done on fresh marrow; thawed marrow is not suitable for this procedure, as the cryopreservant DMSO, even if washed out quickly, is toxic to hematopoietic cells. The thawed marrow should, therefore, be given to the patient immediately.

New marrow purging techniques are being investigated at many centers. These include, for example, immunological methods such as the use of cytokines (e.g., interleukin-2, interferon or tumor necrosis factor) or purging under long-term culture conditions. An important question, however, remains whether relapse is ultimately caused by small numbers of reinfused malignant cells or by malignant clones that have survived high dose chemo/radiotherapy and persist in the patient. Gene marking studies of transplanted cells are currently underway to address this question.

Back-Up Marrow

Ther term "back-up marrow" refers to a fraction of the aspirated marrow which in the case of marrow manipulation remains untreated. The bulk (i.e., about 75%) of the collected marrow undergoes purging and the remainder ($\geq 1 \times 10^8$ nucleated cells/kg) is not treated, but is cryopreserved and stored. If the purged autologous marrow becomes contaminated during processing, or if engraftment is not achieved, this fraction can be used to salvage the patient. However, not all centers routinely collect a back-up marrow, doing so only if new (mostly experimental) techniques are being explored.

Marrow Infusion

Side effects during allogeneic marrow infusion are uncommon. A large-bore central venous catheter should be available; the infusion usually requires about 1–3 hours. Mild hemolysis secondary to ABO-incompatibilities can occur, especially when recipient isoagglutinins are not completely removed by plasma exchange before transplantation. In very small pediatric recipients, marrow infusion may result in volume overload, which can usually be controlled by the administration of diuretics or at times may require apheresis of a corresponding volume of peripheral blood, which can be done manually.

The cryoprotectant (DMSO) used for the storage of autologous marrow can cause nausea, vomiting, flushing, abdominal cramps, chest discomfort and occasional hypotension, apart from the fact that it has an unpleasant odor which may last for about 24 hours. Premedication for the patient usually includes an antinausea drug, an antihistamine and/or hydrocortisone. The bags of marrow are thawed rapidly in a water bath at 37°C and transfused immediately. During marrow infusion, cardiac monitoring is recommended and vital signs should be taken at short intervals. Since DMSO is also toxic to hematopoietic stem cells once the marrow is thawed, the marrow should be given to the patient as quickly as tolerated (usually over 10–30 minutes). DMSO probably also causes mild hemolysis, as most patients after infusion of cryopreserved autologous marrow have a transient elevation of serum lactic dehydrogenase. In severe cases, some form of renal function impairment can be observed.

Other Sources of Stem Cells

Peripheral Blood Stem Cell Transplantation

Hematopoietic progenitor cells capable of repopulating an aplastic marrow circulate in the peripheral blood, albeit at low frequency. These stem cells can be recovered by leukapheresis and reinfused instead of or in addition to bone marrow. This technique is now being used in increasing numbers of autologous transplant recipients. Peripheral stem cell collection is labor-intensive, as it requires staff for repeated leukapheresis and cryopreservation, but has the advantage of not requiring the patient to undergo general anesthesia; this might be of particular value if the donor is at risk for complications due to general anesthesia. Also, some patients with malignant lymphoma may have received irradiation of the pelvis during induction or consolidation treatment, and the yield from pelvic bone may not be sufficient. For these patients, peripheral blood stem cell transplantation may offer a therapeutic option. Some centers consider this technique in patients who have marrow involvement by their disease (e.g., in multiple myeloma). Although malignant cells usually also circulate in blood, their absolute number is considered lower than in marrow and conceivably they are more efficiently removed by purging than is possible with marrow.

Four to eight sessions using a continuous-flow cell separator are usually necessary for stem cell collection. The leukapheresed nucleated cells, which also contain the stem cell fraction, are frozen and stored as described above. The best time to perform an autologous stem cell harvest is usually at the time of "rebound" leukocytosis after chemotherapy; the optimum timing has been determined empirically. The yield might be further increased by the use of hemopoietic growth factors such as granulocyte- (G-) or granulocyte-macrophage (GM-) colony stimulating factor (CSF) given prior to the intended apheresis.

The engraftment kinetics following stem cell transplantation are different from those after marrow transplantation. An initial transient increase of nucleated cells originates from more mature hemopoietic progenitors; this is followed by reconstitution from early pluripotent stem cells. This biphasic pattern can lead to a temporary decline in the neutrophil count, usually between day 20 and 30 after stem cell infusion. A similar kinetic is often observed for platelets; patients who had already been independent of regular platelet transfusions may again become temporarily thrombocytopenic and transfusion-dependent.

Purified Stem Cells

To get closer to the goal of engineering a bone marrow according to the need of the recipient, including the transfer of genes, a major area of research is currently devoted to enrichment procedures to obtain hemopoietic stem cells. Using surface antigen markers (such as CD34) these cells can be enriched by passing the marrow through a column containing the antibody. This marrow can then be further purified for example by using cell sorting of dye labelled marrow cells. Such purified stem cells could be used as targets for gene transfer, either to correct congenital diseases or to introduce drug-resistant genes that would allow only the malignant cells to be killed by chemo/radiotherapy.

Cadaveric Marrow

A cadaveric source of bone marrow is attractive in view of the fact that many patients do not have a suitable living related or unrelated donor. The availability of cadaveric marrow, which must be taken shortly after death and subsequently frozen and stored, might circumvent this shortage. So far, only one case of successful engraftment with cadaveric marrow (father → son) has been reported. The approach seems to be possible; however, further testing and refining is required, particularly in regard to sustained engraftment.

To obtain cadaveric marrow, the outer cortex of both iliac bones is removed with an electrical bone saw, and the trabecular bone marrow containing red marrow can then be extracted using a bone press. Marrow may also be obtained from the lumbar or thoracic vertebrae. Samples are cut into small sections, and stirred with medium for about 30 minutes to release marrow cells. After passing through a stainless steel sieve, the cells are layered over Ficoll-Hypaque to enrich for mononuclear cells and remove debris. The resulting cell suspension is then depleted of T-cells and cryopreserved as described above.

Umbilical Cord Blood Cells

Cord blood contains hemopoietic progenitors. Thus far, two patients with Fanconi's anemia have received successful transplants of stem cells obtained from the umbilical cord blood of HLA-identical siblings. Cord blood collected at birth could be kept available throughout an individual's lifetime. Although appealing, this approach has logistical implications (e.g., storage). Moreover, since cord blood cells represent a "naïve" immune system it is unresolved as to how it would acquire immunities to different diseases. Once these issues have been addressed, cord blood could become a source of stem cells for transplantation.

References

Areman EM, Deeg HJ, Sacher RA (1992) Bone Marrow and Stem Cell Processing: A Manual of Current Techniques, I.A. Davis & Co., Philadelphia

Bell AJ, Hamblin TJ, Oscier DG (1986) Circulating stem cell autografts. Bone Marrow Transplant 1:103

Buckner CD, Clift RA, Sanders JE, Stewart P, Bensinger WI, Doney KC, Sullivan KM, Witherspoon RP, Deeg HJ, Appelbaum FR, Storb R, Thomas ED (1984) Marrow harvesting from normal donors. Blood 64:630

Davis JM, Rowley SD, Braine HG, Piantadosi S, Santos GW (1990) Clinical toxicity of cryopreserved bone marrow graft infusion. Blood 75:781

Gorin NC (1986) Collection, manipulation and freezing of haemopoietic stem cells. Clin Haematol 15:19

Lasky LC, Van Buren N, Weisdorf DJ, Filipovich A, McGlave P, Kersey JH, McCullough J, Ramsay NKC, Blazar BR (1989) Successful allogeneic cryopreserved marrow transplantation. Transfusion 29:182

Thomas ED, Storb R (1970) Technique for human marrow grafting. Blood 36:507

Treleaven JG, Kemshead JT (1985) Removal of tumor cells from bone marrow: An evaluation of the available techniques. Hematol Oncol 3:65

III. Acute Transplant Related Problems

1. Side Effects of Conditioning Regimens

Overview

Despite the reconstitutive effects of marrow transplantation on hematopoiesis, severe hematologic and non-hematologic toxicity is produced by the myeloablative conditioning regimens commonly used to condition patients. Specific toxicities depend on the agents employed, their dose and schedule as well as the patient's overall clinical condition, co-morbid illness, prior treatment, disease status, excretory-organ function, concomitant medications, etc. Disease status is a particularly important prognostic factor for toxicity, as it is a rough but useful gauge of the extent of prior therapy and the resultant degree of organ damage. Moreover, patients with advanced disease status will tend to tolerate therapy less well for other reasons related to the presence of advanced disease.

Severe hematologic toxicity is produced by the marrow ablation that is often, but not always, one goal of the conditioning regimen. Pancytopenia is usually manifest either by the day of transplantation (day 0) or soon afterward, depending to some extent on the underlying disease and the current state of hematopoiesis. The onset also depends upon the specific conditioning regimen used; for example, busulfan (1 mg/kg po q6 h × 4 days) followed by cyclophosphamide (50–60 mg/kg iv daily × 2–4 days) produces a slightly slower and more gradual onset of pancytopenia than do regimens of cyclophosphamide and total body irradiation (TBI) at doses of ≥1000 cGy. In any case, virtually all patients are at risk of neutropenic infection and thrombocytopenic hemorrhage until recovery of the transplanted marrow begins several weeks later. The infective consequences of neutropenia are discussed more fully in III.4.

Table 13. Acute complications of conditioning regimens

- Pancytopenia
- Mucositis and other oral complications
- Nausea and emesis
- Gastroenteritis and diarrhea
- Urotoxicity
- Renal toxicity
- Hepatic damage
- Cutaneous toxicity
- Neurotoxicity
- Cardiotoxicity
- Interstitial pneumonitis
- Fluid and electrolyte imbalance

The situation involving non-hematologic or extramedullary toxicities (listed in Table 13) is different, virtually never being the goal of therapy, and is usually the more serious. Moreover, various non-hematologic organs are damaged not only by the conditioning regimen but also by other post-transplant modalities (e.g., methotrexate, cyclosporine, nephrotoxic antibiotics, etc.), and the extent that these factors contribute to overall toxicity is often difficult to assess precisely. Therefore, regimen-related toxicity is simplest to assess in the situation that requires the lesser amount of post-transplant therapy – autologous marrow transplantation.

Recently, a pragmatic schema attempting to semi-quantify regimen-related toxicity has been proposed (Table 14); in general, $0 =$ none, $1 =$ mild, $2 =$ moderate, responding to therapy, $3 =$ life-threatening, and $4 =$ fatal. Certain of these toxicities appear relatively soon after conditioning is given, while others may manifest later. Note that, according to this schema, the maximal grade is that present at day +28 (with the exception of lung toxicity, which is evaluated up to day +100). Therefore, a patient dying of hepatotoxicity on day +28 would be considered grade IV regimen-related toxicity, while if the patient died one day later on day +29, the maximal grade would only be III! The cumulative regimen-related toxicity score is also occasionally given; such is complicated by the fact that a score of IV in one organ is fatal, while grade I toxicity in four or more organs would likely not be. Despite these shortcomings, this schema should be used, although modifications would be useful.

Only those regimen-related toxicities observed before day +100 will be discussed in this section; later-occurring toxicities are discussed in IV.7.

Specific Complications

These are listed in Table 13. Certain of these complications are discussed in greater detail in III.5–III.8.

Pancytopenia

Pancytopenia and associated infection and hemorrhage are considered in detail in Section III.4.

Mucositis and Other Oral Complications

Most conditioning regimens produce some mucositis, usually during the first few weeks after transplantation. The use of certain agents (e.g., TBI, etoposide, melphalan or thio-TEPA) in conditioning regimens will increase the frequency and severity of mucositis. Also, the use of methotrexate in the acute graft-versus-host disease (GVHD) prophylaxis regimen will produce or aggravate mucositis produced by the conditioning regimen.

While mucositis and other oral complications (such as various infections) are not entirely preventable with current conditioning regimens, other complications may be reduced albeit only to a degree by correcting pre-existing problems such as gingival disease, caries and partially erupted wisdom teeth. If such problems are found, consultation with, and ideally correction by, a dentist or oral surgeon is recommended before initiating the transplant sequence. A regular oral hygiene regimen during the first few weeks after transplantation is also important, although exactly what components are necessary is not clear; chlorhexidine rinses q 4 h during waking hours are commonly used.

Interestingly, the hemorrheologic agent pentoxifylline may be useful in ameliorating mucositis (probably mediated

Table 14. Regimen-related toxicity according to organ system

	Grade I	Grade II	Grade III
Bladder	Macroscopic hematuria after 2 days from last chemotherapy dose with no subjective symptoms of cystitis and not caused by infection	Macroscopic hematuria after 7 days from last chemotherapy dose not caused by infection; or hematuria after 2 days with subjective symptoms of cystitis not caused by infection	Hemorrhagic cystitis with frank blood, necessitating invasive local intervention with installation of sclerosing agents, nephrostomy or other surgical procedure
Cardiac	Mild ECG abnormality, not requiring medical intervention; or noted heart enlargement on chest x-ray with no clinical symptoms	Moderate ECG abnormalities requiring and responding to medical intervention; or requiring continuous monitoring without treatment; or congestive heart failure responsive to digitalis or diuretics	Severe ECG abnormalities with no or only partial response to medical intervention; or heart failure with no or only minor response to medical intervention; or decrease in voltage by more than 50%
CNS	Somnolence but the patient is easily arousable and oriented after arousal	Somnolence with confusion after arousal; or other new objective CNS symptoms with no loss of consciousness not more easily explained by other medication, bleeding or CNS infection	Seizures or coma not explained (documented) by other medication, CNS infection, or bleeding
GI	Watery stools >500 mL but <2000 mL every day, not related to infection	Watery stools ≥2000 mL every day, not related to infection; or macroscopic hemorrhagic stools with no effect on cardiovascular status, not caused by infection; or subileus not related to infection	Ileus requiring nasogastric suction and/or surgery and not related to infection; or hemorrhagic enterocolitis affecting cardiovascular status and requiring transfusion

Hepatic	Mild hepatic dysfunction with bilirubin ≥2.0 mg% and ≤6.0 mg%; or weight gain >2.5% and <5% from baseline, of noncardiac origin; or SGOT increase more than 2-fold but less than 5-fold from lowest preconditioning	Moderate hepatic dysfunction with bilirubin >6 mg% and <20 mg%; or SGOT increase >5-fold from preconditioning; or clinical ascites or image documented ascites >100 mL; or weight gain >5% from baseline of noncardiac origin	Severe hepatic dysfunction with bilirubin ≥20 mg%; or hepatic encephalopathy; or ascites compromising respiratory function
Pulmonary	Dyspnea without chest x-ray changes not caused by infection or congestive heart failure; or chest x-ray showing isolated infiltrate or mild interstitial changes without symptoms not caused by infection or congestive heart failure	Chest x-ray with extensive localized infiltrate or moderate interstitial changes combined with dyspnea and not caused by infection or congestive heart failure; or decreased PO_2 (>10% from baseline) but not requiring mechanical ventilation or >50% O_2 on mask and not caused by infection or congestive heart failure	Interstitial changes requiring mechanical ventilatory support or >50% oxygen on mask and not caused by infection or congestive heart failure
Renal	Increase in creatinine up to twice the baseline value (usually the last recorded before the start of conditioning)	Increase in creatinine above twice baseline but not requiring dialysis	Requirement of dialysis
Stomatitis	Pain and/or ulceration not requiring a continuous IV narcotic drug	Pain and/or ulceration requiring a continuous IV narcotic drug (morphine drip)	Severe ulceration and/or mucositis requiring preventive intubation; or resulting in documented aspiration pneumonia with or without intubation

Note: Grade IV regimen-related toxicity is defined as fatal toxicity.
Adapted from Bearman et al (1988), J Clin Oncol 6: 1562.

via tumor necrosis factor α [TNF-α] inhibition), although more information is needed. Likewise, the use of certain recombinant hematopoietic growth factors (e.g., granulocyte colony-stimulating factor [G-CSF] or granulocyte-macrophage colony-stimulating factor [GM-CSF]) may be helpful by hastening neutrophil recovery, which in turn contributes to healing of the oral mucosa.

When mucositis is first noted, oral feedings and medications should be minimized or discontinued. Cultures should be performed, and treatment begun if a specific infectious agent is identified. As discussed in III.4, acyclovir should generally be used prophylactically in herpes simplex-seropositive patients. Supportive therapy consists of parenteral nutrition and opiate analgesia given by continuous infusion in severe cases.

In any case, the complete or near-complete avoidance of mucositis is an important goal, having significant implications regarding both patient comfort and economics: a major reduction in mucositis would likely reduce the need for a variety of intravenous medications (e.g., opiates, parenteral nutrition) and allow for the substitution of oral (or enteral) nutritive or other agents (e.g., cyclosporine and acyclovir) earlier, and possibly contribute to earlier hospital discharge.

Nausea and Emesis

Although usually limited to a relatively short period of time, peri-conditioning nausea and emesis are not only severely problematic to the patient but also likely increase the later need for the intravenous route of administration of drugs and parenteral nutrition, features that increase the cost of the transplant. While there is general agreement that the vigorous use of various antiemetics (e.g., metoclopramide, diphenhydramine, dimenhydrinate, dexamethasone) is of some benefit – albeit with great individual variation – in reducing nausea produced by the conditioning regimen, side effects such as sedation and the "extrapyramidal syndrome" are common. More recently, a new class of antiemetics, the serotonin antagonists (e.g., ondansetron and granisetron), have been introduced with initial reports indicating an increase in therapeutic efficacy and fewer adverse reactions. If this is confirmed, their use may become routine despite their relatively high cost.

In any case, nausea and emesis usually subside within a few days following conditioning. However, some patients experience prolonged symptoms without (another) obvious etiology. Most will require endoscopy and/or contrast studies to exclude another diagnosis.

Gastroenteritis and Diarrhea

It may be assumed that agents in the conditioning regimen that produce stomatitis will produce mucosal damage throughout the gastrointestinal tract, a common manifestation of which is diarrhea. However, diarrhea may be multifactorial, due to a variety of bacterial and viral infections, acute GVHD or certain medications which may produce or exacerbate diarrhea. Accordingly, these causes should be excluded with appropriate cultures, endoscopy and biopsy. Oral intake should be minimized or discontinued, and the institution of parenteral nutrition considered. Opiates are often helpful for symptomatic control of diarrhea. Finally, the presence of diarrhea is also an indication that oral drug absorption may be unreliable and intravenous medications should be substituted; this applies especially to cyclosporine.

Urotoxicity

As discussed more fully in III.7, the hemorrhagic cystitis that occurs soon after marrow grafting is usually due to acrolein, a urotoxic metabolite of the drug cyclophosphamide (a component of most conditioning regimens), but may occasionally be produced by other agents (e.g., etoposide). It appears to be especially common with the busulfan and cyclophosphamide regimen. Hemorrhagic cystitis usually appears within 2 weeks after cyclophosphamide administration; it can also occur later, but it is uncertain how frequently this is related to secondary causes such as viral infections or, more arguably, even GVHD (see also III.7).

Satisfactory – but not completely effective – prophylaxis usually can be achieved with hyperhydration ($\geq 3.0\,L/m^2/day$), or by using the uroprotective compound mesna (2-mercaptoethane sulfonate sodium) until at least 48 hours after the last cyclophosphamide dose; neither regimen is clearly superior in the usual case, although the optimal schedule for administration of mesna has not yet been fully determined. (This statement regarding mesna applies primarily to cyclophosphamide, but most investigators assume that mesna is also needed for prophylaxis with ifosfamide, an agent much less frequently used in conditioning regimens.) Simple bladder irrigation does not appear to be a useful adjunct.

Relatively mild cases of hemorrhagic cystitis can be managed with additional or continued hyperhydration and/or continuous bladder irrigation. Platelet transfusions to maintain levels above those usually needed for adequate hemostasis (e.g., $30-50 \times 10^9/L$) are useful. Pain is often severe, and analgesia and spasmolytics are indicated. Urethral catheterization and continuous bladder irrigation are especially indicated if the patient is passing large clots, and a variety of methods (including formalin or alum instillation) have been used to control this complication, albeit with variable results. Cystoscopy and cauterization is sometimes helpful; even cystectomy may be needed in rare cases. More recently, prostaglandin instillation has been advocated; results are anecdotal as of this writing. Obviously, urologic consultation is useful for these more severe cases.

As with other complications, successful prophylaxis of hemorrhagic cystitis would be most desirable in reducing the costs of marrow transplantation.

Renal Toxicity

While severe nephrotoxicity directly due to commonly-used conditioning regimens such as cyclophosphamide plus total body irradiation (CY + TBI) or busulfan plus cyclophosphamide (BUCY) is unusual, a degree of renal insufficiency after transplantation is common. Of course, regimens including known nephrotoxins (e.g., cisplatin) will produce more nephrotoxicity. In any case, most cases of abnormal renal function post-transplant are related to (or greatly augmented by) nephrotoxic agents which are not components of the conditioning regimen, specifically cyclosporine, aminoglycosides, amphotericin B, and occasionally acyclovir. Generally, the problem of abnormal renal function can be managed by dose alterations or the use of alternative agents. However, dialysis is occasionally required, almost invariably in patients with abnormal renal function pre-transplant and those receiving cyclosporine.

Interestingly, a clinical picture resembling a "hemolytic-uremic syndrome" (HUS) can be seen after transplants of any type. Although this HUS-like problem is usually seen >6 months post-transplant, it can occasionally be observed earlier. The treatment is as for HUS (i.e., plasma exchange, etc.), although mortality is considerable.

Hepatic Damage

Some degree of hepatotoxicity is common after almost every conditioning regimen, and such often presages the development of serious toxicities in other organs (e.g., the kidneys). Although it usually occurs earlier, hepatic toxicity may be difficult to differentiate from hepatic dysfunction related to GVHD, viral hepatitis or other infections.

The most important regimen-related toxicity is the pathologic lesion of veno-occlusive disease (VOD) of the liver, which is discussed more fully in Section III.6. The usual clinical manifestations of VOD are tender hepatomegaly, fluid retention, weight gain and jaundice, and usually develop within the first 2 weeks post-transplant. VOD is not always predictable, but is more frequent and severe in patients with pre-existing hepatitis, those with extensive prior chemotherapy, those receiving "augmented" conditioning regimens and those receiving allogeneic marrow transplants. Recent evidence also suggests a correlation in certain patients receiving busulfan in the conditioning regimen with pharmacokinetic data and VOD.

Non-invasive tests, especially the hepatic ultrasonogram, are generally not diagnostic but may be helpful in excluding other etiologies. The hepatic artery resistive index, obtained by duplex sonograph, may be more useful. Liver biopsy may be needed, and should be undertaken (possibly via the transvenous route).

Prophylaxis, therapy and prognosis of VOD are discussed in III.6.

In addition to VOD, other hepatic lesions are associated with some conditioning regimens. High doses of carmustine, for example, or occasionally even cyclophosphamide and TBI, can result in hepatic necrosis.

Cutaneous Toxicity and Alopecia

While cyclophosphamide often produces a transient rash, severe cutaneous toxicity is only rarely due to the conditioning regimen. However, toxic erythema can be seen following the use of high-dose cytarabine or thio-TEPA. Also, radiation recall dermatitis may occur and occasionally be severe. The optimal prophylaxis or therapy for these problems is unknown; however, topical and even systemic steroids may be useful in some cases.

Capital alopecia tends to be total, while loss of body hair is more variable. This complication is usually wholly (if slowly) reversible. However, exceptions do occur, especially with the use of busulfan and cyclophosphamide conditioning, and regrowth of hair may be incomplete in patients with chronic GVHD of the skin.

Neurotoxicity

Although technically not components of the conditioning regimen, the use of intrathecal chemotherapy immediately before and sometimes following conditioning can produce a myriad of complications; these are beyond the scope of this discussion but are discussed more fully in III.8.

Leukoencephalopathy is one of the most serious neurological complications that develop post-transplant, but is usually a chronic rather than an acute disorder and occurs infrequently (see Section III.8). Serious acute complications due to high-dose chemotherapy elements include cerebellar toxicity with high-dose cytarabine regimens, seizures with high-dose busulfan and peripheral neuropathy as well as ototoxicity with high-dose carboplatin. Neurotoxicity due to cytarabine can be prevented somewhat by limiting the use of high-dose cytarabine regimens to younger patients and, by inference from chemotherapy studies, by using single and cumulative doses less than $3 g/m^2$ and $36 g/m^2$, respectively. Moreover, patients who have had cerebellar toxicity due to prior high-dose cytarabine should not receive this agent in the conditioning regimen, even if resolution has been complete. Effective levels of phenytoin can also reduce seizures produced by busulfan, but require determination by serum assay.

Although they are not well documented, unexplained polyneuropathies can be observed in the post-transplant setting. It is unclear whether these are a side-effect of conditioning or related to other post-transplant problems such as GVHD.

Extrapyramidal reactions are often noted with certain antiemetics, but are not due to the conditioning regimen per se; they are usually readily reversible by dose modification or diphenhydramine. Also, cyclosporine may cause a variety of neurologic problems such as cortical blindness, seizures, tremor and encephalopathy; these are discussed in III.8.

Cardiotoxicity

Cardiotoxicity, if it occurs, is usually manifest a few days following high doses of cyclophosphamide (>200 mg/kg), and presents clinically as a hemorrhagic peri-myocarditis of high lethality. Therefore, all calculations for cyclophosphamide should be made on the basis of ideal body weight, or at least adjusted ideal body weight. Moreover, the traditional method of giving cyclophosphamide (as daily doses over several hours) is being re-examined; some centers use a twice-daily or a continuous administration schedule. While it is unclear whether cardiomyopathy is more common in patients with pre-existing heart disease due to organic or therapy-related causes, alternatives to the use of cyclophosphamide (e.g., melphalan or antithymocyte globulin) should at least be considered in this circumstance.

Interstitial Pneumonitis

Interstitial pneumonitis is discussed more fully in III.5. This term does not relate to a specific disease but rather a clinical, radiographic and histologically-defined syndrome. The best characterized cases of interstitial pneumonitis are infectious in origin, often due to cytomegalovirus. However, conditioning (especially when involving TBI) is felt to influence the process denoted as "idiopathic" interstitial pneumonitis; fractionated TBI reduces the incidence of this complication considerably. Of particular note, idiopathic interstitial pneumonitis is found with increased frequency in patients who had previously received significant amounts of thoracic or mediastinal radiotherapy and were given TBI-containing conditioning; alternative (i.e., non-TBI) conditioning should thus be chosen when possible in such patients.

While there is no specific treatment, some investigators use high-dose steroids with variable but generally unsatisfactory results; the use of intravenous pentoxifylline is currently being explored. Conversely, for patients with diffuse alveolar hemorrhage, a problem which may mimic interstitial pneumonitis and which is noted especially in autologous transplant patients, a short course of high-dose corticosteroids may be useful.

Although carmustine (BCNU) is not a usual component of conditioning regimens for allogeneic marrow transplantation, it is used more often in autotransplant regimens for leukemia, lymphoma and breast cancer. When used in this manner, BCNU can produce an acute interstitial pneumonitis; it is thought that prior mediastinal irradiation or prior nitrosourea use increases the probability of this complication. The recognition of this problem, and its prompt treatment with high-dose steroids, may be lifesaving; bronchoalveolar lavage and possibly open lung biopsy should be performed promptly to exclude an infective process.

Fluid and Electrolyte Imbalance

Given the copious quantities of intravenous medications (including intravenous nutrients) required for virtually all marrow transplant patients, the fluid shifts associated with VOD, the nephrotoxicity and electrolyte loss associated with certain antibiotics and cyclosporine, the complex metabolic problems of prolonged corticosteroid use, and the secondary diarrhea associated with GVHD, it is not surprising that problems of fluid and electrolytes arise soon after marrow transplantation. However, these problems are, in general, generic to very ill patients, and are rarely difficult to correct provided that close monitoring and prompt intervention are carried out.

The capillary leak syndrome, often associated with general fluid retention, can occur in patients around the time of marrow engraftment; some transplant physicians consider it a symptom of "hyperacute" GVHD. Symptoms include rapidly deteriorating respiration with concomitant drop in oxygen saturation and arterial oxygen concentration. Some patients may require ventilatory support.

The syndrome is believed to be caused by a massive release of cytokines (such as TNF-α and various interleukins), which is known to disrupt interepithelial adhesion and allow fluid to enter the interstitial lung space. The capillary leak syndrome occurs predominantly in patients who have received a transplant from a non-histocompatible sibling or unrelated donor. It is variably responsive to higher doses of steroids, diuretics, and, if the serum level is decreased, albumin infusions.

Future Directions

It is helpful to define a group of patients at high risk of developing regimen-related toxicity; perhaps the routine use of pharmacokinetics will be more useful than certain clinical characteristics, allowing such measures as intra-treatment dose adjustment as is now being done in some centers for busulfan. (However, the overall value of such is not fully proven.)

Nevertheless, there are circumstances in which the propensity to regimen-related toxicity will be unknown or unavoidable, and some general method to ameliorate such toxicity would be extremely helpful, both in reducing the level of toxicity from current regimens and in potentially allowing for the safe use of further-intensified conditioning. Although no standard regimen currently exists, it is likely that a variety of "protective" agents will be utilized including various cytokines (e.g., hematopoietic growth factors) and inhibitors of cytokine action (e.g., pentoxifylline), as well as other agents designated to counter toxic effects on specific organ systems.

However, the available agents are not optimal, and while a reduction in regimen-related toxicity is highly desirable in the interim, this goal may be difficult to achieve without a decrement in intensity – and therefore a loss of efficacy of conditioning, since there is a rough correlation between efficacy and toxicity of conditioning regimens. A simpler, if not completely effective approach to toxicity reduction is by earlier transplantation whenever possible, since this minimizes the possibility of cumulative toxicity from prior therapy.

References

Atkinson K, Biggs JC, Golovsky D, Concannon A, Dodds A, Downs K, Ashby M (1991) Bladder irrigation does not prevent haemorrhagic cystitis in bone marrow transplant recipients. Bone Marrow Transplant 7:351

Baker BW, Wilson CL, Davis AL, Spearing RL, Hart DNJ, Heatin DC, Beard MEJ (1991) Busulphan/cyclophosphamide conditioning for bone marrow transplantation may lead to failure of hair regrowth. Bone Marrow Transplant 7:43

Bearman SI, Appelbaum FR, Buckner CD, Petersen FB, Fisher LD, Clift RA, Thomas ED (1988) Regimen-related toxicity in patients undergoing bone marrow transplantation. J Clin Oncol 6:1562

Bearman SI, Appelbaum FR, Back A, Petersen FB, Buckner CD, Sullivan KM, Schoch HG, Fisher LD, Thomas ED (1989) Regimen-related toxicity and early posttransplant survival in patients undergoing marrow transplantation for lymphoma. J Clin Oncol 7:1288

Bianco JA, Appelbaum FR, Nemunaitis J, Almgren J, Andrews F, Kettner P, Shields A, Singer JW (1991) Phase I–II trial of pentoxifylline for the prevention of transplant-related toxicities following bone marrow transplantation. Blood 78:1205

Braverman AC, Antin JH, Plappert MT, Cook EF, Lee RT (1991) Cyclophosphamide cardiotoxicity in bone marrow transplantation: A prospective evaluation of new dosing regimens. J Clin Oncol 9:1215

Chao NJ, Duncan SR, Long GD, Horning SJ, Blume KG (1991) Corticosteroid therapy for diffuse alveolar hemorrhage in autologous bone marrow transplant recipients. Ann Intern Med 114:145

Deeg HJ, Spitzer TR, Cottler-Fox M, Cahill R, Pickle LW (1991) Conditioning-related toxicity and acute graft-versus-host disease in patients given methotrexate/cyclosporine prophylaxis. Bone Marrow Transplant 7:193

Gottdiener JS, Appelbaum FR, Ferrans VJ, Deisseroth A, Ziegler J (1981) Cardiotoxicity associated with high-dose cyclophosphamide therapy. Arch Intern Med 141:758

Grigg AP, Shepherd JD, Phillips GL (1989) Busulphan and phenytoin. Ann Intern Med 111:1049 [Correction in: Ann Intern Med 112:313 (1990)]

Grochow LB, Jones RJ, Brundrett RB, Braine HG, Chen T-L, Saral R, Santos GW, Colvin OM (1989) Pharmacokinetics of busulfan: Correlation with veno-occlusive disease in patients undergoing bone marrow transplantation. Cancer Chemother Pharmacol 25:55

Herbetko J, Grigg A, Buckley AR, Phillips GL (in press) Veno-occlusive liver disease after bone marrow transplantation: Findings at duplex sonograph. AJR Am J Roentgenol

Jones RJ, Lee KSK, Beschorner WE, Vogel VG, Grochow LB, Braine HG, Vogelsang GB, Sensenbrenner LL, Santos GW, Saral R (1987) Venoocclusive disease of the liver following bone marrow transplantation. Transplantation 44:778

Juckett M, Perry EH, Daniels BS, Weisdorf DJ (1991) Hemolytic uremic syndrome following bone marrow transplantation. Bone Marrow Transplant 7:405

Nevill TJ, Barnett MJ, Klingemann H-G, Reece DE, Shepherd JD, Phillips GL (1991) Regimen-related toxicity of a busulfan-cyclophosphamide conditioning regimen in 70 patients undergoing allogeneic bone marrow transplantation. J Clin Oncol 9:1224

Pecego R, Hill R, Appelbaum FR, Amos D, Buckner CD, Fefer A, Thomas ED (1986) Interstitial pneumonitis following autologous bone marrow transplantation. Transplantation 42:515

Powles R, Pedrazzini A, Crofts M, Clink H, Millar J, Bhattia G, Perez D (1984) Mismatched family bone marrow transplantation. Semin Hematol 21:182

Shepherd JD, Pringle LE, Barnett MJ, Klingemann H-G, Reece DE, Phillips GL (1991) Mesna versus hyperhydration for the prevention of cyclophosphamide-induced hemorrhagic cystitis in bone marrow transplantation. J Clin Oncol 9:2016

Szeluga DJ, Stuart RK, Brookmeyer R, Utermohlen V, Santos GW (1987) Nutritional support of bone marrow transplant recipients: A prospective, randomized clinical trial comparing total parenteral nutrition to an enteral feeding program. Cancer Res 47:3309

Weiner RS, Bortin MM, Gale RP, Gluckman E, Kay HEM, Kolb H-J, Hartz AJ, Rimm AA (1986) Interstitial pneumonitis after bone marrow transplantation: Assessment of risk factors. Ann Intern Med 104:168

2. Acute Graft-Versus-Host Disease (GVHD)

With a successful marrow transplant, the recipient's lympho-hemopoietic cells are replaced by donor-derived cells. Thus, in contrast to solid organ transplantation where the recipient's immune system remains in place and attempts at immunosuppression are aimed at preventing the reaction of recipient cells against the transplanted organ, a double-barrier exists in marrow transplantation: transplanted marrow may fail to reconstitute successfully hemopoiesis in the recipient (graft failure due to immunological mechanisms or other factors) or donor lymphocytes may attack recipient tissue. While graft failure has generally been a problem only with HLA incompatible transplants, after marrow T-cell depletion and in some patients sensitized by prior transfusions, GVHD has been a major problem with all allogeneic transplants. We have to assume that in all instances of marrow transplantation an interaction between donor and host cells (graft-vs-host reaction) takes place. However, it was noted in early experiments that syngeneic, i.e., genetically identical marrow, could be transferred to a pretreated recipient without any clinically recognizable adverse reaction. In contrast, when marrow from an allogeneic donor was used a clinical syndrome developed which was originally termed secondary disease. This syndrome, subsequently called GVHD, is manifested mostly in skin, liver, and intestinal tract, although other targets such as the conjunctivae can be involved as well (see Table 15).

Mechanisms of GVHD

Early experimental studies suggested that the development of GVHD was closely related to the administration of immuno-

Table 15. Targets of acute GVHD

Skin
Liver
Intestinal Tract
Oral Mucosa
Conjunctivae
Airways (?)
Exocrine glands (?)

competent lymphocytes from the marrow donor. There was evidence that increasing the number of lymphoid cells increased the likelihood, and shortened the time interval to the development of acute GVHD. In 1966, Billingham summarized the essential requirements for the development of GVHD as follows:

a) the graft must contain immunologically competent cells;
b) the recipient must express relevant transplantation antigens that are not present in the donor, and consequently are capable of immunologically stimulating donor cells;
c) the recipient must be immunologically deficient, i.e., incapable of mounting an immune response that would result in the destruction of transferred donor cells.

It is clear that these requirements are met not only after allogeneic marrow transplantation but also after the transplantation of solid organs that contain lymphoid tissue and after transfusion of non-irradiated blood products, particularly in neonates, in patients with congenital immunodeficiencies and in patients receiving radiochemotherapy.

Finally, under certain clinical conditions GVH reactions can occur between genetically identical individuals (monozygotic twins) or even after autologous marrow infusion. These observations have necessitated, therefore, a revision of Billingham's second postulate to include the inappropriate recognition of self antigens.

GVHD is currently understood as an immunopathophysiologic process with two consecutive phases. The recipient tissues first activate T lymphocytes from the donor (afferent phase); the activated T cells then secrete cytokines, recruit additional cells, induce the expression of histocompatibility antigens, and focus the attack of donor effector cells on recipient targets (efferent phase).

Acute GVHD

The afferent phase of acute GVHD can be considered in three steps: antigen presentation, activation of individual T cells, and proliferation and differentiation of activated T cells. During antigen presentation, proteins are digested by antigen-presenting cells into smaller fragments and these antigenic peptides bind to HLA (Class I or II) molecules and are displayed on the surface of the antigen-presenting cells as peptide-HLA complexes. T cells recognize this complex through antigen-specific T-cell receptors. In allogeneic interactions such as GVHD, mature donor T cells recognize recipient peptide-HLA complexes (alloantigens), in which either the HLA molecules or the bound peptides are foreign. The host antigen-presenting cells release cytokines, including a second activation signal required for naive T cells, interleukin-1. In addition to the T-cell receptor, accessory molecules such as CD4, CD8, CD44, and lymphocyte function antigens (LFA-1 and LFA-2) participate in interactions between effectors and target cells.

Antigen presentation induces the second step, the activation of individual T cells. This involves numerous intracellular biochemical changes, including an increase in cytoplasmic free calcium and activation of protein kinase C and tyrosine kinases. These pathways then activate the transcription of genes for cytokines, e.g., interleukin-2, and their receptors. Interleukin-2 stimulates the proliferation of cells that secrete it (autocrine effect) and of other cells expressing the receptor (paracrine effect).

The third step involves clonal expansion and differentiation. Cells then produce proteins required for specific effector functions. This differentiation is accompanied by alteration of numerous cell surface molecules.

The alloantigens of the host determine which subset of T cells proliferates and differentiates. Differences in MHC Class

II molecules (HLA-DR, DP, and DQ) stimulate CD4+ T cells, and differences in MHC Class I molecules (HLA-A, B, and C) stimulate CD8+ T cells. In mouse models of GVHD, in which genetic differences between donor and recipient can be controlled, CD4+ T cells induce GVHD in response to MHC Class II antigen differences, and CD8+ T cells induce GVHD in response to MHC Class I antigen differences. It appears that in HLA identical marrow transplants, GVHD can be induced by either subset or simultaneously by both.

The efferent arm of acute GVHD is less well understood. Recent experimental data emphasize the role of soluble mediators (cytokines), in particular, tumor necrosis fact or α, an inflammatory cytokine that has been shown in mice to be a central mediator of GVHD. Tumor necrosis factor is released by T cells and large granular lymphocytes or macrophages after stimulation by other cytokines and directly or indirectly results in cytolysis.

It is controversial whether in man large granular lymphocytes or natural killer cells induce the changes that occur after the T-cell-mediated GVH reaction. The precise relation between cytokines and secondary effector cells must still be clarified. These interactions are further complicated by the presence of natural suppressor cells. It may become possible to use cytokines to alter imbalances of these networks and to promote tolerance. For example, experimental data show that interleukin-2 given to mice with some delay after transplantation may exacerbate GVHD, whereas when given immediately post-transplant can reduce mortality from acute GVHD by 70 percent.

Chronic GVHD

Chronic GVHD is discussed in detail below (IV.2). It is important to note here that patients with acute GVHD, even Grade I, are more likely to develop chronic GVHD than patients who never had acute GVHD. However, even without preceding acute GVHD de novo chronic GVHD can develop.

Syngeneic GVHD

Pathological changes resembling GVHD have been observed in irradiated and cyclosporine-treated animals that have received marrow from genetically identical donors (or even autologous marrow). Clinically, GVHD after transplantation in identical twins was described more than a decade ago. Syngeneic GVHD appears to be mediated by autoreactive lymphocytes directed at MHC Class II proteins. These autoreactive T cells escape the usual negative selection (clonal deletion) within the damaged thymus. This escape is enhanced by the administration of cyclosporine, and autoreactive T cells migrate to the periphery, where they trigger or mediate damage to the target organ. Other regulatory lymphocytes, which could inactivate such autoreactive cells, have been eliminated by total-body irradiation as part of the preparative regimen. The effects of cyclosporine are important in these models, both in preventing the reestablishment of regulatory cells and in allowing the development of autoreactive cells; these two processes seem related to the damage that cyclosporine inflicts on the thymic medulla. Syngeneic GVHD can thus be seen as an imbalance between autoreactive and autoregulatory lymphocytes.

Clinical Features of Acute GVHD

Acute GVHD in man usually develops within 2–8 weeks of marrow transplantation. The main target organs are listed in Table 15. There is no universal agreement as to how GVHD should best be graded. Although the criteria originally proposed by the Seattle group continue to form the basis of all grading systems (Fig. 2), some modifications appear indicated.

GVHD can present as a hyperacute syndrome and clinical findings of severe inflammation with high fever and capillary damage with extravasation and fluid retention. These features, which at times may be difficult to distinguish from conditioning related toxicity (III.1), can develop within 4 or 5 days of transplantation and have been observed especially in patients not given post-grafting immunosuppression or transplanted

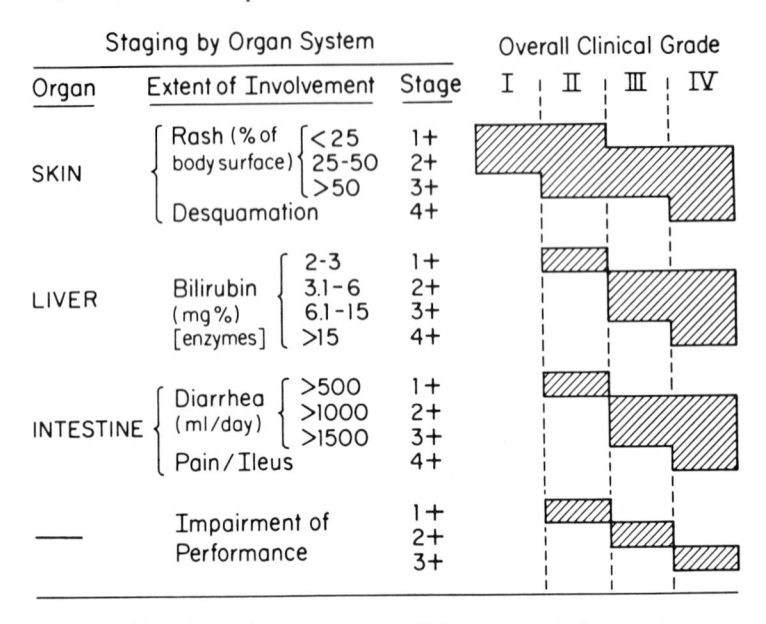

Staging by Organ System			Overall Clinical Grade
Organ	Extent of Involvement	Stage	I | II | III | IV
SKIN	Rash (% of body surface) <25 / 25-50 / >50; Desquamation	1+ / 2+ / 3+ / 4+	
LIVER	Bilirubin (mg%) [enzymes] 2-3 / 3.1-6 / 6.1-15 / >15	1+ / 2+ / 3+ / 4+	
INTESTINE	Diarrhea (ml/day) >500 / >1000 / >1500; Pain/Ileus	1+ / 2+ / 3+ / 4+	
—	Impairment of Performance	1+ / 2+ / 3+	

Fig. 2. Clinical grading of acute GVHD. The left panel of the figure summarizes the grading by organ system; the right panel shows the overall clinical grade. With grade I, only the skin can be involved. With more extensive involvement of the skin or involvement of liver and intestinal tract and impairment of the clinical performance status, either alone or in any combination, the severity grade advances from II to IV. (Reprinted with permission from H.J. Deeg et al., "Graft-versus-host disease: Pathophysiological and clinical aspects", Ann Rev Med 1984; 35:11–24

with marrow from an HLA nonidentical donor. Usually, these findings are not reflected in the commonly used grading scheme. This also applies to patients with nausea or vomiting without other gastrointestinal manifestations. Similarly, patients may show only mild bilirubin abnormalities but marked transaminase elevations, thought to represent hepatic GVHD. On the other hand, hepatic GVHD is difficult or impossible to assess if another hepatic complication, in particular veno-occlusive disease is present.

Generally, however, the onset of acute GVHD is marked by a maculo-papular rash involving face, palms and soles, subsequently spreading and possibly involving the entire body (Fig. 3). Bullae may ensue, and the patient may have the appearance of a total body burn. Concurrently or subsequently,

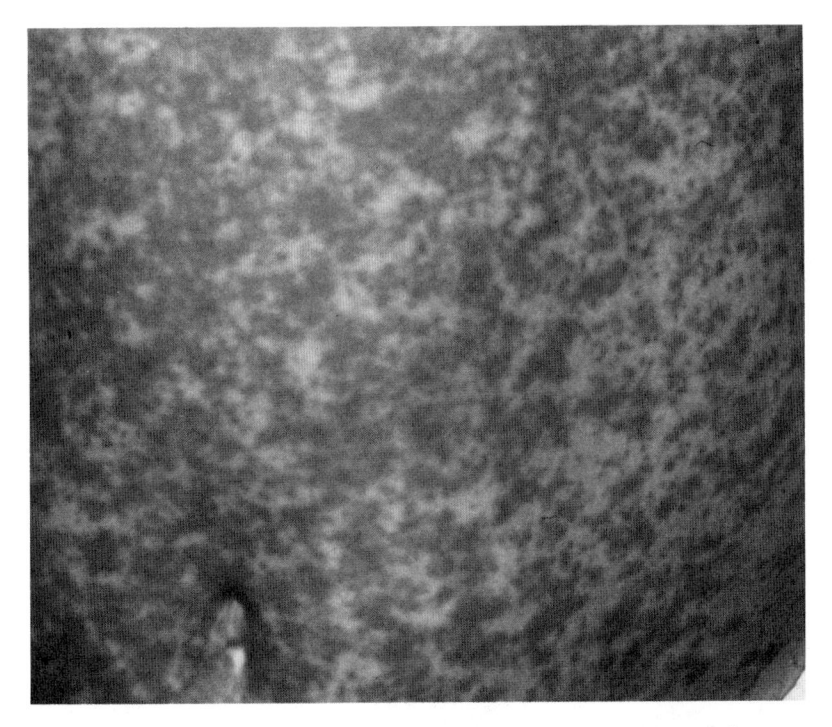

Fig. 3. Acute GVHD of the skin with diffuse erythema and superimposed maculopapular eruption and associated edema of the dermis

Table 16. Diagnosis of acute GVHD

Clinical Picture (Skin, Liver, Intestinal Tract)
Skin Biopsy
Rectal Biopsy
Chemistry Survey
Radiograph of the Abdomen
(Gastric or Duodenal Biopsy)
(Liver Biopsy)

the bilirubin may rise along with an elevation of serum alkaline phosphatase and aspartate aminotransferase. There may also be nausea and vomiting along with watery, often greenish stained or bloody diarrhea, and abdominal pain.

Some GVHD diagnostic procedures are listed in Table 16. The radiographic appearance of the intestinal tract is illustrated

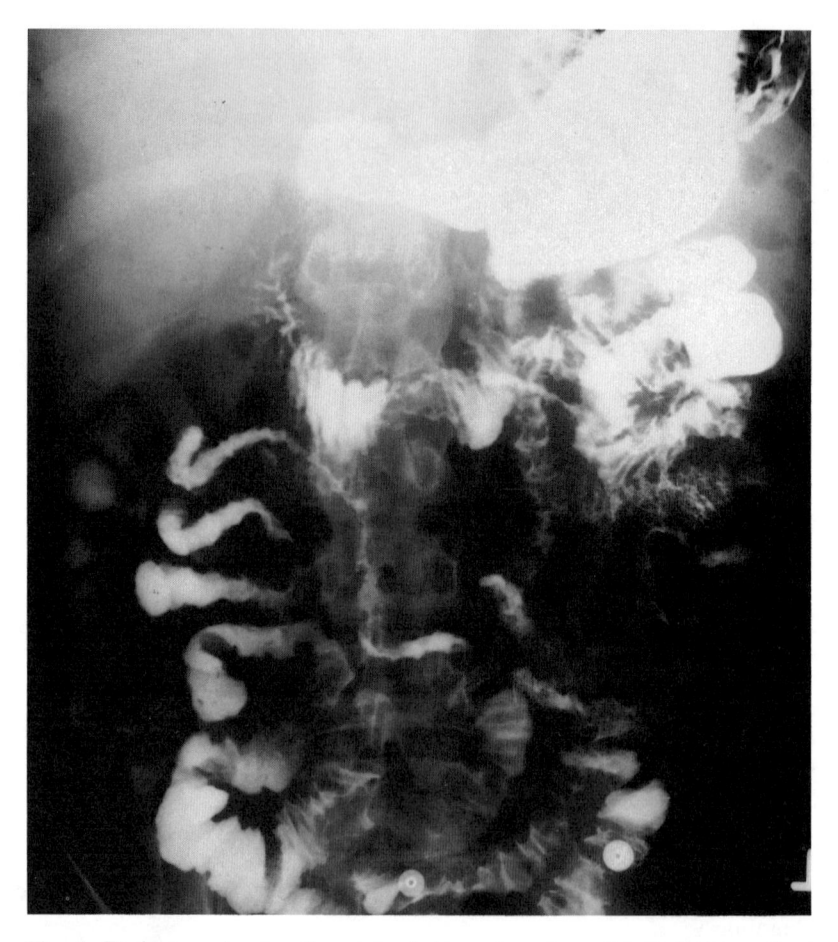

Fig. 4. Barium contrast radiograph of stomach and small bowel of a patient with acute GVHD. Stomach and duodenum are normal in appearance. There is edema of the bowel wall from mid-jejunum to terminal ileum with luminal narrowing, thumbprinting, and separation of adjacent loops (courtesy of G. McDonald, M.D.)

by Fig. 4. The histological alterations have been described elsewhere. Although only a rare patient will die from causes *directly* related to acute GVHD, 5–10% of patients will succumb to associated complications. Infections are frequent during the first 3–4 months and are described in detail below.

Table 17. Timing of GVHD prophylaxis

Donor treatment before marrow aspiration
Marrow manipulation in vitro
Recipient treatment
– before marrow transplant
– after marrow transplant

Prevention of GVHD with Drugs

From the earlier discussion it is clear that several options for GVHD prevention are available; these are schematically summarized in Table 17. Conceivably, one could treat the marrow, which is to be transplanted, while it still resides in the prospective marrow donor. Studies in rodent models suggest that antisera or monoclonal antibodies directed at T lymphocytes, at large granular lymphocytes or their precursors in the donor or PUVA treatment of the donor may have a beneficial effect for the prevention of GVHD in the prospective recipient. Only one clinical study has been reported to date. Jacobs and coworkers treated prospective marrow donors with cyclosporine for 2 weeks before marrow aspiration and transplantation into the recipient. In this small uncontrolled study no advantage to this approach was noted.

Most clinical studies have used post transplantation treatment of the recipient with immunosuppressive agents. Until recently the two most widely applied regimens involved small doses of methotrexate (10 or 15 mg/m^2) or cyclophosphamide given intermittently for approximately three months after transplantation. This approach resulted in a 35–50% incidence of acute GVHD. In the late 1970's cyclosporine became available. Cyclosporine is usually given on a daily basis starting one day before marrow infusion and continued for variable periods of time after transplantation, generally ranging from 3–12 months. With the oral preparation of the drug, doses have ranged from 10–25 mg/kg, generally around 12 mg/kg/day. Three randomized studies have been reported comparing methotrexate with cyclosporine in patients with hematologic malignancies. The incidence of acute GVHD of grades II-IV ranged from 19–57% in patients given methotrexate, and from 40–56% in patients given cyclosporine. Overall there was no significant difference or advantage for either one of the two drugs.

Since even with prophylactic measures as many as 50% of patients developed acute GVHD, some investigators questioned whether these agents had any beneficial effect and embarked upon studies omitting post-grafting immunosuppression. An additional argument in favor of these studies was the possibility that the omission of GVHD prophylaxis might result in a desirable graft-versus-leukemia effect. One such study revealed a comparable incidence of GVHD for patients given methotrexate and patients given no postgrafting prophylaxis. Another study comparing, in sequential fashion, a standard course of methotrexate as described above with a short course of methotrexate, given on days 1 to 6, found a similar (60–70%) incidence of GVHD. A third study in patients less than 30 years of age, and transplanted from HLA identical donors, observed a 25% incidence of acute GVHD with a standard course of methotrexate, 61% with a short course of methotrexate and 100% without post grafting immunosuppression. Most investigators now agree that no allogeneic transplant should be carried out without GVHD prophylaxis.

The usefulness of postgrafting immunosuppression is further substantiated by recent trials using combinations of drugs. One study at the University of Minnesota, using a combination of methotrexate, prednisone, and antithymocyte globulin (ATG) showed an incidence of acute GVHD of 21% compared to 48% in a control group given methotrexate only. Studies at the Fred Hutchinson Cancer Research Centers in Seattle comparing cyclosporine and methotrexate given alone as compared to a combination of cyclosporine plus methotrexate found an incidence of acute GVHD of 28% in patients given the cyclosporine combination. A study at Johns Hopkins University in Baltimore, comparing cyclosporine plus prednisone to cyclophosphamide plus prednisone found a significant reduction of GVHD from 68% to 32% using the cyclosporine combination. Similar results have been reported from numerous institutions world wide.

While these regimens have reduced the incidence of acute GVHD, morbidity still is substantial in those who develop the syndrome. Since particularly in patients transplanted for non-malignant disease no benefit in the form of a graft-versus-leukemia effect can be expected, studies have been designed to prevent GVHD even more effectively. In one trial methotrexate was given at doses of $10\,mg/m^2$ on days 1, 3 and 6 only in combination with continuous infusion cyclosporine and intermittent high doses of intravenous immunoglobulin, resulting in a 10% incidence of acute GVHD with HLA identical transplants.

In another trial prednisone was added to methotrexate and cyclosporine, beginning on day 0. Surprisingly, the incidence of GVHD with prednisone was higher than without prednisone, conceivably because prednisone interfered with the action of methotrexate. The probability of relapse, on the other hand, was lower with the addition of prednisone, possibly due to a direct effect of prednisone or because of an increased graft-versus-leukemia effect associated with more GVHD. The latter would be consistent with the observation in numerous studies indicating a higher probability of leukemic relapse, in particular in patients with acute myelogenous leukemia, with improved GVHD prevention.

The incidence of acute GVHD is substantially higher in patients transplanted from HLA nonidentical donors, reaching 80–90% with haplotype different related or phenotypically matched unrelated donors. It was of note, however, that survival was not proportionally decreased, presumably due to different graft/host interactions resulting in a more profound graft-versus-leukemia effect and a lower probability of relapse than seen in HLA identical transplant recipients. GVHD was increased especially in those patients in whom a mismatch existed in the GVH direction and less so in those with a difference in the HVG direction.

T-Cell Depletion

Following the recognition in animal models that T lymphocytes played an essential role in the initiation of GVHD, studies were carried out to test this hypothesis. Indeed, it could be shown that mice transplanted with T lymphocyte depleted marrow across major histocompatibility barriers did not develop GVHD, and reconstituted to become completely immunocompetent chimeras. Similar studies have been reported in dogs and monkeys. Based on that information clinical trials were initiated.

Initially Rodt and coworkers used a heteroantiserum directed at human lymphocytes to incubate donor marrow cells before infusion into the recipient. No source of complement was added under the assumption that opsonization of T lymphocytes would result in their rapid removal by the patient's reticuloendothelial system. Among 20 patients, only six developed signs of GVHD. It was of note, however, that 2 patients failed to achieve engraftment. With the arrival of monoclonal antibodies directed at specific subpopulations of human cells, individual antibodies, or combinations thereof, have been used to manipulate marrow. Mouse monoclonal antibodies with pan-T specificity (cluster of differentiation [CD]3, CD5 etc.) or with specificities directed at subpopulations of T cells, (e.g., CD8), have generally been used in conjunction with rabbit complement to eliminate the relevant cells in vitro before infusion into the recipient. This approach has been applied with both HLA identical and nonidentical transplants. Studies are too numerous to be listed individually, but results can be summarized as follows: Effective depletion of T lymphocytes (3–4 logs) results in a reduced incidence of acute and probably chronic GVHD. Concurrently with the reduction of GVHD, however, several problems were noted. While patients given unmanipulated marrow from an HLA identical sibling donor almost uniformly achieve sustained engraftment, (with graft failure being observed in only 1–2% of patients), 10–40% of patient experienced graft failure with marrow depleted of T cells by monoclonal antibodies and complement. The incidence of graft failure was even higher with T cell depleted marrow from HLA nonidentical donors. Some investigators have argued that failure of engraftment was only due to insufficient immunosuppression of the recipient. Conceivably, the complete or partial elimination of immunocompetent donor T lymphocytes not only eliminated the effector cells of GVHD, but also cells with anti-host reactivity necessary for optimum engraftment. Hence, the effect otherwise mediated by donor T lymphocytes would have to be achieved by other means, e.g., additional immunosuppression. If this speculation is correct, however, it would also point the way towards alternative approaches in the form of more selective inhibition of host cells, thereby avoiding increased toxicity otherwise associated with broader and more aggressive immunosuppression of the recipient. Experimental approaches currently being investigated include the use of immunotoxin conjugates or radioactive isotope-coupled monoclonal antibodies directed at recipient immune and marrow cells.

In patients who achieve engraftment, immunoreconstitution proceeds at a rate comparable to that seen in patients given unmanipulated marrow. For some patient populations, such as children with SCID, in whom graft failure is not a problem, T cell depleted marrow transplantation is the treatment of choice. For patients with other disorders, especially with nonmalignant hemopoietic diseases such as severe aplastic anemia, the risk of non-engraftment has to be weighed against that associated with the development of GVHD.

Of note is the development of rat antihuman monoclonal antibodies which activate human complement and, hence, are not dependent upon an exogenous source of complement. The most widely used antibody is Campath 1, a broadly reactive antibody which recognizes the majority of human T cells, B cells, and some NK cells. Several hundred transplants from HLA identical donors using this approach have been reported. Less than 10% of these patients developed clinically relevant acute GVHD. However, similar to studies using murine monoclonal antibodies, 15–20% of patients given HLA identical marrow graft failed to achieve sustained engraftment.

In part due to the concern about unreliability of complement sources, investigators have searched for means of

T cell elimination that do not depend upon complement. Pioneered by Reisner and coworkers a method combining the use of soybean agglutination and rosette formation with sheep red blood cells is used effectively at Sloan Kettering Memorial Cancer Center, to eliminate T cells from donor marrow. A disadvantage of this method is that it is very time intensive; an advantage may be a somewhat lower incidence of graft-failure.

Another method employs magnetic biospheres to which monoclonal antibodies have been coupled. The antibodies will attach to the relevant cells which in turn are removed by passage through a magnetic field. This method is currently used successfully to eliminate tumor cells from autologous marrow. Some investigators feel that it may also be a superior method for T cell depletion. Another approach is the coupling of monoclonal antibodies to immunotoxins, e.g., ricin A chain or diphtheria toxin. Following the binding of the antibody to the relevant cell, the toxin molecule enters the cell and destroys it. Using methods of molecular biology this approach has recently been further refined by generating hybrid molecules which deliver the toxin even more reliably to the target cell. The method of counter flow elutriation, in principal a sophisticated modification of gradient techniques uses different centrifugal force and flow rates (rather than densities) to separate different cell populations from each other. Centers in Europe and in the United States have reported very encouraging results with this method. Contrary to some of the studies using monoclonal antibody and complement, failure of engraftment does not appear to be a problem. This might be due to the fact that a substantial number of T lymphocytes is still being infused. Available data suggest that approximately 10^5 lymphocytes/kg may be acceptable in regards to GVHD prevention and sufficient to ensure engraftment. Other efforts have included chemoseparation using agents such as methylprednisolone, for preincubation of donor marrow. Although quite promising in rodent models, preliminary clinical data have been disappointing.

In addition to graft failure, a second disturbing finding in patients given T cell depleted marrow grafts was the rather high incidence of disease recurrence. In patients with chronic myelogenous leukemia given Campath I treated marrow grafts the probability of disease recurrence ranged from 40–70%; in some patients transplanted at an advanced stage of their disease the probability of relapse approached 100%. In retrospect this may not be surprising. Studies in rodent models had shown that animals with leukemia that developed GVHD had a lower relapse rate of leukemia than recipients without GVHD. This has been attributed to a termed graft-vs-leukemia effect. Analyses of several clinical marrow transplant trials have also shown that patients with acute or chronic GVHD or both have a better chance of remaining in remission than patients without GVHD. It is thought that the graft-vs-leukemia effect is also mediated by T lymphocytes.

So far it has not been possible to separate a graft-vs-leukemia effect from GVHD, even though there are data suggesting a beneficial allogeneic effect in patients who do not develop GVHD as indicated by a lower incidence of leukemic relapse than in patients transplanted from a syngeneic donor. A recent study suggests, nevertheless, that a measurable graft-vs-leukemia effect occurred only in patients with clinically manifest GVHD but not in those with subclinical GVHD. Currently ongoing studies explore the usefulness of the administration of Interleukin-2 (Il-2) or Il-2 plus LAK cells in reducing the incidence of leukemia relapse. This post-transplant immunotherapy may mimic a graft-vs-leukemia effect, and these patients may show clinical signs reminiscent of GVHD.

The Effect of a Germ-Free Environment (Gnotobiosis) on GVHD

The approach of transplanting patients in a germfree environment along with skin and gastrointestinal decontamination is rather attractive, although logistically quite involved and expensive. Conceptually this approach prevents T cell activation by eliminating microbial antigens that may cross-react with antigens of the patient or cause non-specific activation of antigen presenting cells. The responses of T cells via their receptors to "superantigens" such as staphylococcus enterotoxin

Table 18. Agents for prevention and treatment of GVHD

In vivo	In vivo or in vitro	In vitro
Methotrexate Cyclophosphamide Azathioprine 6-mercaptopurine Procarbazine Cyclosporine FK506 Anti-thymocyte globulin (ATG) Thalidomide Immunoglobulin Pentoxifyllin Gnotobiosis	Glucocorticoids Monoclonal antibodies Immunotoxins Phototherapy	Elutriation Soybean and sheep red blood cell agglutination

might explain such a phenomenon. In addition gnotobiosis may reduce the production of endotoxin and result in an effect similar to that observed recently with the blockade of tumor necrosis factor α.

To date positive results have been reported only in patients with nonmalignant diseases, i.e., patients conditioned with chemotherapy alone, rather than regimens including the use of TBI. Presumably, patients given only chemotherapy had less gastrointestinal toxicity and were able to comply with the administration of oral nonabsorbable antibiotics, resulting in decontamination sufficient to have an impact on the prevention of GVHD. In patients given TBI, compliance was poor, decontamination was less successful, and consequently, GVHD developed.

Treatment of GVHD

Methods used clinically for prophylaxis and treatment of GVHD are listed in Table 18. The drugs listed are generally more effective for prophylaxis than for therapy, presumably because fewer cells have been activated and fewer secondary signals and cell populations have been triggered. This is important since different interventions may be desirable at different stages.

Glucocorticoids are considered standard therapy. Generally, methylprednisolone is given i.v. at 2 mg/kg/day in divided doses. Approximately 30–50% of patients respond completely or partially. At higher doses, 4 or even 20 mg/kg/day, the response rate may increase; however, generally experience has shown that overall outcome is not improved, mainly because of a high incidence of infection. Less frequently this approach has been complicated by pancreatitis and, with some delay, aseptic necrosis of the bone.

ATG has induced responses in 25–30% of patients with acute GVHD. Monoclonal antibodies, either unmodified or coupled to toxins (e.g., ricin A chain conjugated to an anti-CD5 antibody) have been used in numerous investigations, but their exact place in the therapy of acute GVHD remains to be determined. Other agents including cyclosporine, either alone or in combination with ATG or glucocorticoids offer useful therapy in patients who have not received cyclosporine as part of a prophylactic regimen.

A recent analysis by Martin and colleagues suggests that overall only 20% of patients achieve a complete response to initial therapy. This is important since completeness of response correlates with the probability of long-term survival. Response of established GVHD to therapy does not negate an antileukemic effect of GVHD.

Recent developments include the production of humanized versions of murine monoclonal antibodies (e.g., against the IL-2 receptor) which, because of different pharmacokinetics and lack of immunogenicity are expected to provide better anti-GVHD therapy. Other agents, listed in Table 18 (FK506, thalidomide, phototherapy, etc.) or not listed (rapamycin, succinyl acetone, etc.), are currently being tested in clinical and experimental trials.

References

Atkinson K, Horowitz MM, Gale RP, Van Bekkum DW, Gluckman E, Good RA, Jacobsen N, Kolb H-J, Rimm AA, Ringdén O, Rozman C, Sobocinski KA, Zwaan FE, Bortin MM (1990) Risk factors for chronic graft-versus-host disease after HLA-identical sibling bone marrow transplantation. Blood 75:2459–2464

Burakoff SJ, Deeg HJ, Ferrara J, Atkinson K (1990) Graft-vs-Host Disease: Immunology, Pathophysiology, and Treatment. Marcel Dekker Inc. New York 1–725

Champlin R, Ho W, Gajewski J, Feig S, Burnison M, Holley G, Greenberg P, Lee K, Schmid I, Giorgi J, Yam P, Petz L, Winston D, Warner N, Reichert T (1990) Selective depletion of CD8+ T lymphocytes for prevention of graft-versus-host disease after allogeneic bone marrow transplantation. Blood 76:418–423

Deeg HJ, Henslee-Downey PJ (1990) Management of acute graft-versus-host disease. Bone Marrow Transplantation 6:1–8

Deeg HJ, Cottler-Fox M (1990) Clinical spectrum and pathophysiology of acute graft-vs.-host disease. In: Burakoff SJ, Deeg HJ, Ferrara J, Atkinson K (eds): Graft-vs-Host Disease: Immunology, Pathophysiology, and Treatment. Marcel Dekker, New York 311–335

Ferrara JLM, Deeg HJ (1991) Graft-versus-host disease. N Engl J Med 324:667–674

Glucksberg H, Storb R, Fefer A, Buckner CD, Neiman PE, Clift RA, Lerner KG, Thomas ED (1974) Clinical manifestations of graft-versus-host disease in human recipients of marrow from HL-A-matched sibling donors. Transplantation 18:295–304

Korngold R, Sprent J (1978) Lethal graft-versus-host disease after bone marrow transplantation across minor histocompatibility barriers in mice. Prevention by removing mature T cells from marrow. J Exp Med 148:1687

Lazarus HM, Coccia PF, Herzig RH, Graham-Pole J, Gross S, Strandjord S, Gordon E, Cheung NKV, Warkentin PI, Spitzer TR, Warm SE (1984) Incidence of acute graft-versus-host disease with and without methotrexate prophylaxis in allogeneic bone marrow transplant patients. Blood 64:215

Maraninchi D, Mawas C, Guyotat D, Reiffers J, Vernant JP, Gratecos N, Hirn J, Novakovitch G (1988) Selective depletion of marrow-T cytotoxic lymphocytes (CD8) in the prevention of graft-versus-host disease after allogeneic bone-marrow transplantation. Transplant Int 1:91–94

Martin PJ, Kernan NA (1990) T-cell depletion for the prevention of graft-vs.-host disease. In: Burakoff SJ, Deeg HJ, Ferrara J, Atkinson K (eds), Graft Versus Host Disease: Immunology, Pathophysiology, and Treatment. Marcel Dekker, New York 371–387

Mitsuyasu RT, Champlin RE, Gale RP, Ho WG, Lenarsky C, Winston D, Selch M, Elashoff R, Giorgi JV, Wells J, Terasaki P, Billing R, Feig S (1986) Treatment of donor bone marrow with monoclonal anti-T-cell antibody and complement for the prevention of graft-versus-host disease. Ann Intern Med 105:20–26

Rappeport J, Mihm M, Reinherz E, Lopansri S, Parkman R (1979) Acute graft-versus-host disease in recipients of bone marrow transplants from identical twin donors. The Lancet II, 717

Ringden O, Bäckman L, Tollemar J, Heimdahl A, Aschan J, Gahrton G, Ljungman P, Lönnqvist B, Sundberg B (1989) Long-term follow-up of a randomized trial comparing graft-versus-host disease prophylaxis using cyclosporin or methotrexate in patients with haematological malignancies. Bone Marrow Transplantation 4(Suppl. 2):119

Sale GE, Shulman HM (1984) The pathology of bone marrow transplantation. Masson Publishing, New York

Schattenberg A, De Witte T, Preijers F, Raemaekers J, Muus P, Van Der Lely N, Boezeman J, Wessels J, Van Dijk B, Hoogenhout J, Haanen C (1990) Allogeneic bone marrow transplantation for leukemia with marrow grafts depleted of lymphocytes by counterflow centrifugation. Blood 75:1356–1363

Storb R, Deeg HJ, Pepe M, Doney K, Appelbaum F, Beatty P, Bensinger W, Buckner CD, Clift R, Hansen J, Hill R, Longton G, Anasetti C, Martin P, Loughran TP, Sanders J, Singer J, Stewart P, Sullivan KM, Witherspoon R, Thomas ED (1989) Graft-versus-host disease prevention by methotrexate combined with cyclosporin compared to methotrexate alone in patients given marrow grafts for severe aplastic anaemia: Long-term follow-up of a controlled trial. Br J Haematol 72:567–572

Storb R, Pepe M, Anasetti C, Appelbaum FR, Beatty P, Doney K, Martin P, Stewart P, Sullivan KM, Witherspoon R, Bensinger W, Buckner CD, Clift R, Hansen J, Longton G, Loughran T, Petersen FB, Singer J, Sanders J, Thomas ED (1990) What role for prednisone in prevention of acute graft-versus-host disease in patients undergoing marrow transplants? Blood 76:1037–1045

Vossen JM, Heidt PJ, Guiot HFL, Dooren LJ (1981) Prevention of acute graft versus host disease in clinical bone marrow transplantation: complete versus selective intestingal decontamination. S. Sasaki et al. (eds), Recent Advances in Germfree Research, Tokai University Press 573

Wagner JE, Santos GW, Noga SJ, Rowley SD, Davis J, Vogelsang GB, Farmer ER, Zehnbauer BA, Saral R, Donnenberg AD (1990) Bone marrow graft engineering by counterflow centrifugal elutriation: Results of a phase I–II clinical trial. Blood 75:1370

3. Marrow Graft Failure

To achieve sustained marrow engraftment the patient's own immune cells must be eliminated or suppressed in order to allow donor-derived cells to replace the patient's lympho-hemopoietic system. Under controlled experimental conditions it is possible to distinguish between graft rejection due to a memory response following preceding sensitization, and failure of sustained engraftment in a nonsensitized recipient on the basis of genetic (hybrid, allogeneic) resistance. It is more difficult to separate these two mechanisms in man. Sometimes it is not certain whether a patient has been transfused or not, sometimes transfusions are given in the peri-transplant period, i.e. while the patient is receiving immunosuppressive therapy. Furthermore, factors other than allosensitization and resistance, e.g., defects of the microenvironment, can contribute to graft failure. In any event graft failure can manifest itself either as primary engraftment failure or as initial engraftment followed by secondary graft loss, generally within weeks, occasionally later. Graft failure may or may not be associated with reappearance of recipient cells, i.e. there may be cellular and occasionally humoral evidence of a host response to the attempted graft, or the graft may be lost for other reasons without there ever being an active host response. The latter certainly applies in patients given autologous grafts.

The definition of graft failure has been somewhat controversial. Generally, however, if a patient's granulocyte count is not sustained at $>200/\mu l$ by day 21 or, at the latest, day 28, graft failure is thought to be present. The diagnosis is further substantiated by biopsy findings of an empty marrow or low marrow cellularity without the presence of identifiable myeloid, erythroid or megakaryocytic precursors.

Some tests for documentation of donor cell engraftment are

Table 19. Documentation of donor cell engraftment

Cytogenetic analysis of metaphase spreads
(Constitutive or after stimulation)
– Sex chromosome
– Autosomal chromosome marker
HLA Typing[a]
– Serological
– Restriction fragment length polymorphism (RFLP)
– Sequence – specific oligonucleotide probes (SSOP)
Complement typing
Immunoglobulin allotyping
Erythrocyte typing[b] – Antigens
– Enzymes

[a] Especially helpful with HLA non-identical transplants; however, polymorphic DNA sequences outside HLA can be recognized by RFLP, SSOP or other probes.
[b] Currently used only infrequently.

listed in Table 19. In some instances transplant recipients become "mixed chimeras", a term referring to the fact that these patients carry normal lymphohemopoietic cells of donor and host origin. These cell mixtures may persist for years and possibly for the patient's entire life.

The mechanisms involved in graft failure are incompletely understood; however, at least five categories can be distinguished:

a) In the presensitized patient given HLA identical unmanipulated marrow
b) In the patient transplanted with histoincompatible marrow
c) In the patient transplanted with T cell depleted marrow
d) In the patient transplanted with autologous marrow
e) In the patient with marrow defects.

The Presensitized Patient

Animal studies predicted that a transplant recipient given transfusions before transplantation would be at increased risk of rejecting a marrow graft even from a histocompatible donor. This was indeed the case in patients with aplastic anemia. Patients who had been multiply transfused before marrow transplantation and who were conditioned with cyclophosphamide alone (without the use of TBI) in preparation for marrow transplantation for aplastic anemia had a probability of 30–60% of rejecting a graft from an HLA genotypically identical brother or sister, whereas only 5% of untransfused patients given the same conditioning regimen were found to reject their marrow graft. Experimental results suggested that graft rejection was due to sensitization of the recipient to minor histocompatibility antigens, presumably shared between transfusion donor and marrow donor and not expressed on recipient cells. Exposure to those same antigens at the time of transplantation, therefore, elicited a secondary immune response which is more difficult to suppress with conventional methods than a primary immune response encountered in nonsensitized patients.

Different approaches have been taken to overcome this problem. Based on studies in a dog model the Seattle group added the infusion of viable peripheral blood leukocytes from the marrow donor to the marrow inoculum. This approach has reduced the probability of rejection to approximately 5–10%, i.e., to a level not different from that seen in untransfused patients, who, however, were given bone marrow only and no additional peripheral blood leukocytes. This difference is important since the infusion of viable donor leukocytes is associated with a higher risk of GVHD, especially chronic GVHD, than seen without leukocyte infusion. Consequently regimens that ensure engraftment without this side effect would be desirable.

Experience in patients who had rejected their initial graft indicated that a combination of cyclophosphamide (4×50 mg/kg) and ATG (3×30 mg/kg) allowed for sustained engraftment in the majority of evaluable patients. Since regimen-related toxicity was low, such a regimen was attractive for conditioning patients for their first graft, thereby eliminating hopefully the need for donor leukocyte infusions. A currently ongoing study is encouraging in so far as 29 of 30 patients so treated achieved sustained engraftment; the incidence of GVHD appears to be as expected with the use of bone marrow only (R. Storb, personal communication). Other transplant teams have elected to overcome sensitization by increased immunosuppression, usually in the form of drugs or irradiation. Thus, the use of 300 cGy of TBI, or 750 cGy of total lymphoid irradiation (i.e., using radiation protocols similar to those used for the treatment of Hodgkin disease, albeit to a lower total dose), or in a modified form given as thoracoabdominal irradiation in addition to cyclophosphamide, were successful in overcoming rejection. However, this approach seems to be associated with are increased probability of developing a malignant tumor (projected 22% at 10 years) as compared to patients given cyclophosphamide (approximately 6% with follow-up extending to 20 years).

These studies indicate that a patient with aplastic anemia, if possible at all, should be transplanted while still untransfused. Therefore, the physician who evaluates such a patient initially must be aware of these data, and assuming a potential marrow donor is available, should try to avoid transfusion. A transplant center should be contacted immediately for consultation and recommendations in regards to the timing of transplantation and the need for transfusions. Only if the patient is actively bleeding, or requires surgery or some other intervention or shows neurological symptoms suggesting a bleed, should platelet transfusions be given before the situation can be assessed completely. Clinical data indicate that there may be a "window" of approximately 48–72 hours prior to the initiation of the conditioning regimen for transplantation during which transfusions can be given to the patient without jeopardizing the subsequent marrow graft.

Recent reports suggest that it may become possible to transfuse a patient without the risk of sensitization. Studies in dogs have shown that irradiation of blood from the marrow donor with ultraviolet light or gamma irradiation prior to transfusion abrogates the blood's sensitizing ability, and dogs so treated achieve sustained engraftment just as do dogs who have never been transfused. Similarly, dogs given ultraviolet-irradiated platelets from histoincompatible donors are at a significantly lower risk of becoming sensitized and refractory to platelet transfusions than dogs given untreated platelets. There are also preliminary clinical data to suggest that aggressive leukocyte depletion of the transfusion product substantially reduces the risk of sensitization. Leukocytes with antigen presenting ability, such as monocytes, and even more so dendritic cells, appear to be responsible for sensitization.

Pretransplant transfusions in patients with lymphohemopoietic malignancies are apparently not associated with an increased risk of marrow graft rejection. Presumably this is due to the more aggressive cytotoxic therapy, generally involving the use of TBI, that is often employed to prepare these patients for transplantation. Furthermore, in these patients transfusions are generally required because of chemotherapy-induced myelosuppression. This chemotherapy also has immunosuppressive effects, possibly preventing the patient's immune system from responding to the alloantigeneic challenge.

Histoincompatible Transplants

Except in patients with severe aplastic anemia, marrow graft rejection or failure of engraftment of unmanipulated marrow has not been a problem with HLA genotypically identical marrow grafts. However, as more histoincompatible transplants have been carried out, evidence has accumulated that doses of 850–1500 cGy of TBI may be insufficient to suppress the recipient's immune response against major histocompatibility antigens. Even with HLA phenotypically identical marrow from a related donor 6–8% of patients experience graft failure; with marrow differing for 2 or 3 HLA antigens as many as 15 or 20% of patients may fail to achieve sustained engraftment.

As described above, graft failure can occur either in the form of primary failure of engraftment, or with initial evidence of engraftment followed by delayed graft loss. In some respects, these observations resemble those made in animals, especially mice and dogs, showing the phenomenon of genetic resistance. This term generally refers to failure of sustained engraftment of histoincompatible marrow in a setting where major histocompatibility complex matched marrow easily engrafts. However, it is known, again mostly from studies in dogs, that even MHC genotypically identical marrow may not engraft consistently if the intensity of the conditioning regimen is reduced (e.g., 800 cGy in dogs given marrow from a DLA identical donor). Thus, allogeneic resistance is often defined as failure of achieving sustained engraftment after otherwise lethal conditioning.

Since patients given histoincompatible grafts are more likely to develop GVHD and to have more severe manifestations of GVHD than patients transplanted with HLA genotypically identical marrow, they represent a main target group for aggressive attempts at GVHD prevention. Consequently T cell depletion has been tested widely in these patients. Unfortunately, T cell depletion further aggravates the problem of resistance, presumably because the balance between donor and recipient is shifted in favor of the recipient. Approaches to overcome this problem have included the use of increased doses of TBI, or the addition of chemotherapy such as cytosine arabinoside, to regimens consisting of cyclophosphamide and TBI, or the use of monoclonal antibodies and ATG. Clearly, intensified immunosuppression facilitates engraftment; at the same time, however, regimen-related toxicity (intestinal, pulmonary, hepatic) is increased.

Interesting results have been obtained in a canine model with the infusion of monoclonal antibodies directed at class II histocompatibility antigens (MAB 7.2) or at the homing receptor (MAB S5; CD44) in addition to a standard dose of TBI (9.2 Gy). This approach allowed for sustained engraftment in a large proportion of dogs, who with TBI alone almost uniformly fail to engraft. Initial clinical trails with an antibody directed at lymphocyte function antigen I (LFA I) suggest that such an approach might also be feasible and successful in patients.

Other investigators have begun to use monoclonal antibody – conjugated radioisotopes to deliver "in situ" irradiation to leukemia or other malignant cells without causing unacceptable systemic toxicity. A similar approach could possibly be taken to target those cells that mediate resistance to marrow grafts.

T-Cell Depletion

Allogeneic marrow transplantation offers curative therapy for many patients suffering from acute or chronic leukemia, aplastic anemia, or congenital disorders. GVHD contributes substantially to morbidity and mortality associated with this approach even if the transplant is carried out from a genotypically HLA identical donor. Clinically significant acute GVHD is observed in 35-50% of patients given single agent methotrexate, cyclosporine, or cyclophosphamide as post grafting immunosuppressive prophylaxis. Approximately 30-50% of patients develop chronic GVHD; the incidence is particularly high in older patients and in those with preceding acute GVHD. Even with regimens combining agents such as cyclosporine and methotrexate, or cyclosporine and methylprednisolone an incidence of acute GVHD in the range of 20-30% in adult patients has been reported. The incidence of chronic GVHD is similar to that seen with single agents. With HLA nonidentical transplants, dependent upon the degree of mismatch, as many as 60-90% of recipients are expected to develop significant acute GVHD.

Animal models have shown that mature donor T lymphocytes are responsible for triggering GVHD after transplantation of allogeneic marrow or spleen cells. If the marrow is taken from animals that are devoid of mature T-Cells, or if T cells are removed, GVHD can be prevented. Only very few T lymphocytes are necessary to trigger GVHD, even if the transplant is carried out in major histocompatibility complex identical animals i.e., in animals differing only for the so called minor antigens.

On this basis, removal of T lymphocytes from human marrow was attempted as an approach to GVHD. The first attempts involved the use of a heteroantiserum generated in rabbits against human T lymphocytes. Subsequently, fractionation of marrow cells by means of agglutination with lectin, especially soybean agglutinin, and with sheep erythrocytes was achieved. Some studies have used physical methods. Most recent attempts, however, have focused on the use of monoclonal antibodies produced in mice or rats, and directed at specific surface molecules expressed on human T lymphocytes. All studies involving monoclonal antibodies have shown that the use of an exogenous source of complement, or of the donor's own autologous complement in the case of some rat monoclonal antibodies is necessary for treatment success. Alternatives include the coupling of monoclonal antibodies to biomagnetic spheres, allowing for magnetic removal of target cells, or the use of immunotoxins (e.g., coupling of the A chain of ricin to an appropriate monoclonal antibody), which destroy the cells directly. Methods used to remove T lymphocytes in man are summarized in Table 12. The rationale for this approach is that only mature T cells induce GVHD. Thus, if mature cells are removed, T cells developing from lymphohemopoietic stem cells, in a repetition of ontogeny, will differentiate and accept the new (patient) environment as "self", i.e., become tolerant.

In agreement with experimental data, T cell depletion of human marrow significantly reduces the incidence of acute and chronic GVHD. However, along with the very encouraging finding of reduced or absent acute GVHD several rather disturbing observations were made.

The first was failure of sustained engraftment. Failure of engraftment or rejection in patients with a malignant disorder given TBI and an HLA genotypically identical marrow graft is highly unusual (1–2%) without in vitro treatment. With T cell depleted marrow, graft failure has been observed in 15–35% of patients given HLA identical and 30–60% in patients given HLA nonidentical transplants. It is thought that in this setting marrow graft rejection (or non-acceptance), unlike that observed in patients with aplastic anemia who were transfusion-sensitized prior to transplantation, is largely unrelated to pretransplant transfusions. Experimental results in mice and dogs have explained failure of engraftment in non-sensitized recipients on the basis of genetic resistance. Resistance is apparently mediated by antigens outside but linked to the major histocompatibility complex. Resistance can be overcome by more profound immunosuppression of the recipients or by measures directed more specifically at recipient cells involved in resistance. Regardless of the mechanism, these data imply that the presence of T lymphocytes in the marrow graft may have an immunosuppressive effect, either directly, or via the induction of a graft-vs-host reaction, which then might generate the milieu necessary for sustained engraftment. Alternatively, T lymphocytes may have an amplifier effect on transplanted hemopoietic stem cells, thus generating a growth advantage for host cells and leading to "take over" of the host. In response to these observations, the trend has been to intensify immunosuppressive regimens used for conditioning which is effective but carries the risk of increased regimen-related toxicity (see III.1). Attempts at second marrow transplants have almost uniformly been unsuccessful, either due to toxic side effects or to repeated failure of engraftment. It is important, therefore, to monitor not only a patient's blood counts, but also attempt to determine the origin of cells by cytogenetic analysis, or by now available molecular tools to ascertain that engraftment is sustained.

Other modalities are being developed. One group has had considerable success with partial T cell depletion ($\approx 99\%$) combined with in vivo administration of an immunotoxin (Xomazyme $CD5^+$): even with HLA nonidentical transplants engraftment was achieved and GVHD prevented in many instances. Others have carried out T subset ($CD8^+$) depletion of marrow and reported engraftment with a reduced incidence of GVHD. Also counterflow elutriation treated marrow appears to carry a lower risk of resulting in graft failure.

Autologous Marrow Grafts

As outlined elsewhere, autologous transplantation, i.e. the use of the patient's own marrow for reconstitution of lympho-hemopoietic function is being used with increasing frequency and success. There are basically three prerequisites for the feasibility of an autologous transplant:
– It must be possible to obtain sufficiently large numbers of hemopoietic stem (or early precursor) cells capable of self replication and differentiation, and maintenance of viability of these cells.

- The stem (precursor) cell preparation used for infusion should be free of clonogenic tumor cells.
- The patient's malignancy must be responsive to chemoradiotherapy usually given in supralethal doses in preparation for marrow transplantation. (This point, of course, applies not only to autologous, but also to allogeneic transplantation).

Stem cells obtained from the patient's bone marrow (or, for that purpose, from peripheral blood) have generally been exposed to chemotherapeutic regimens, irradiation or both given during initial treatment. Thus they have possibly suffered damage that might impair their ability to reconstitute hemopoietic function after transplantation. There is experimental and clinical evidence that the yield of stem cells, and possibly the quality, depends upon the time point following chemoradiotherapy at which cells are harvested. Dependent upon the agents used for chemotherapy, colony forming units are increased in peripheral blood at a certain time after institution of chemotherapy. The rate of hemopoietic recovery in the autologous setting, although variable, generally appears to depend upon the number of colony forming units (as an indirect assay for hemopoietic precursor cells) transplanted. Accordingly, if small numbers of cells are transplanted or if the cells were harvested after aggressive pretreatment, hemopoietic reconstitution may be protracted or incomplete, at times resulting in death from hemorrhage. "Defective" stem cells seem to be a problem especially in patients with AML.

To obtain the largest possible number of marrow cells is even more important when in vitro manipulation is considered since this usually results in cell loss. The techniques available for autologous "marrow purging" are described above.

Finally, marrow or peripheral blood stem cells harvested for autologous transplantation, must generally be cryopreserved in liquid nitrogen until later use. Cryopreservation may damage any cells, and stem cells in particular. Generally, the approach has been to obtain a large number of cells, such that a loss incurred during cryopreservation would be compensated for. It has been shown that even marrow cryopreserved for 5–10 years can be used successfully for autologous reconstitution after marrow ablative therapy of patients.

However, there still are occasional patients who have incomplete reconstitution of hemopoiesis. Many transplant teams have established a policy, that a second back-up marrow be stored and maintained unmanipulated to serve for rescue should the first transplant (purged in vitro) be unsuccessful (see II.2).

Several areas of ongoing investigation are of interest. Hemopoietic stem cells circulating in peripheral blood have been shown to be capable of complete hemopoietic reconstitution in animal models. These observations have now been confirmed in man, and the data suggest that reconstitution occurs faster than with marrow cells; the rate can be further accelerated if the patient is pretreated with recombinant growth factor (e.g., G-CSF) before the cells are harvested (II.2).

The search for hemopoietic stem cells has resulted in the characterization of very early hemopoietic precursors, for example characterized by antigen CD34, and autologous transplants with positively selected CD34 expressing cells have met with success.

Hemopoietic growth factors (G-CSF, GM-CSF, Il-1, Il-3 etc.) given after autologous or allogeneic transplantation have been shown in several trials to shorten the time period of pancytopenia, and in a proportion of patients, appear to be able to overcome graft failure. The exact place for each of these factors in marrow transplantation remains to be determined.

Other Marrow Defects

Marrow graft failure has been observed in settings that do not fit the above categories. It was noted in patients with severe aplastic anemia that marrow infusions from an identical (syngeneic) twin donor without conditioning of the patient were successful in only half of the patients. Since no genetic differences exist in this setting, other mechanisms, such as autoimmune effects or microenvironmental defects must be invoked. Most but not all of these patients achieved a sustained graft following conditioning and a second marrow infusion.

Observations in allogeneic transplant recipients also suggest additional causes for graft failure. Infection of stromal cells with cytomegalovirus or administration of the antiviral agent gancyclovir, clearly impair hemopoiesis. GVHD may exert an effect directed at the marrow microenvironment leading to the apparent paradox of having GVHD without having achieved a (hemopoietic) graft. Cells may have an altered pattern of cytokine production, and other, ill defined, stromal defects have been reported. Further investigations in this area are required.

References

Anasetti C, Amos D, Beatty PG, Martin PJ, Thomas ED, Hansen JA (1989) Risk factors for graft rejection of marrow transplants from HLA-haploidentical donors. In: Dupont B (ed), Immunobiology of HLA, Vol. II: Immunogenetics and Histocompatibility, Proceedings of the 10th International Histocompatibility Conference. Springer-Verlag, New York 516–517

Barge AJ, Johnson G, Witherspoon R, Torok-Storb B (1989) Antibody-mediated marrow failure after allogenic bone marrow transplantation. Blood 74:1477–1480

Blazar BR, Filipovich AH, Kersey JH, Uckun FM, Ramsay NKC, MacGlave PB, Vallera DA (1987) T-cell depletion of donor marrow grafts: Effects on graft-versus-host disease and engraftment. Progress in Bone Marrow Transplantation. Gale RP and Champlin R (eds), Alan R Liss 381

Cheson BD, lacerna L, Leyland-Jones B, Sarosy G, Wittes RE (1989) Autologous bone marrow transplantation. Current status and future directions. Ann Intern Med 110:51–65

Deeg HJ, Self S, Storb R, Doney K, Appelbaum FR, Witherspoon RP, Sullivan KM, Sheehan K, Sanders J, Mickelson E, Thomas ED (1986) Decreased incidence of marrow graft rejection in patients with severe aplastic anemia: Changing impact of risk factors. Blood 68:1363–1368

Gluckman E, Horowitz MM, Champlin RE, Hows JM, Bacigalupo A, Biggs JC, Camitta BM, Gale RP, Gordon-Smith EC, Marmont AM, Masaoka T, Ramsay NKC, Rimm AA, Rozman C, Sobocinski A, Speck B, Bortin MM (1992) Bone marrow transplantation for severe aplastic anemia: influence of conditioning and graft-versus-host disease prophylaxis regimens on outcome. Blood 79:269–275

Kernan NA (1990) Graft failure following transplantation of T-cell depleted marrow. Burakoff SJ et al. (eds), Graft-vs-Host Disease: Immunology, Pathophysiology, and Treatment. Marcel Dekker, New York 557–568

Reiffers J, Bernard P, David B, Vezon G, Sarrat A, Marit G, Moulinier J, Broustet A (1986) Successful autologous transplantation with peripheral blood hemopoietic cells in a patient with acute leukemia. Exp Hematol 14:312–315

Simmons P, Kaushansky K, Torok-Storb B (1990) Mechanisms of a cytomegalovirus-mediated myelosuppression: Perturbation of stromal cell function versus direct infection of myeloid cells. Proc Natl Acad Sci USA 87:1386–1390

Storb R, Deeg HJ (1986) Failure of allogeneic canine marrow grafts after total-body irradiation. Allogeneic "resistance" versus transfusion-induced sensitization. Transplantation 42:571–575

4. Management of Infections

Overview

A wide variety of common and uncommon infective organisms, including bacterial, fungal, viral and protozoal species, produce major complications after marrow transplantation. While the management of the main categories of infectious problems encountered is discussed below, specific details regarding various therapeutic maneuvers (especially doses and schedules of various anti-infective agents) should be obtained from source materials.

Following myeloablative therapy and marrow transplantation, patients endure an obligate period of severe pancytopenia. Although usually limited to a few weeks, some patients have persistent or recurrent pancytopenia, usually but not always due to inadequate engraftment. Moreover, most marrow transplant recipients also have concomitant disruption of mucosal surfaces and indwelling intravenous lines, and all have significant suppression of humoral and cellular immunity for some months after transplantation. In addition, allogeneic marrow transplant patients often develop graft-versus-host disease (GVHD); this process and its therapies (e.g., corticosteroids, anti-thymocyte globulin, etc.) are additionally immunosuppressive. It is therefore not surprising that complicating infections are both frequent and severe in the marrow transplant setting, beginning early and persisting for some time after the transplant.

Principles of Infection Management

Several principles are fundamental to the general approach to infection in the transplant setting:

1. All infections are potentially serious. As a corollary, evidence of possible infection (e.g., certain clinical signs, positive surveillance cultures, "contaminants" in various cultures, etc.) should not be disregarded without full consideration of its potential importance;
2. Definite diagnosis is critical; if simpler diagnostic methods are not available, tissue for diagnosis should be obtained promptly, both to permit accurate prognosis and especially to select specific therapy (which is often more toxic in the post-transplant setting);
3. Treatment for an infection should be started promptly, empirically if necessary, and in full dose; therapeutic modifications may be made according to response and/or subsequent data;
4. Attempts to reverse underlying complications such as pre-existing infections, graft failure and GVHD are essential.

Donor Considerations

The history of prior infections in the marrow donor is important. For example, a spectrum of infections including cytomegalovirus (CMV), malaria, hepatitis B and human immunodeficiency virus (HIV) have been transmitted in some cases via the marrow (or other donated blood products). A history of such infections may complicate or even contraindicate marrow donation: for example, a CMV-negative patient with more than one otherwise-suitable donor should usually have a seronegative donor chosen, if other factors are equal. Moreover, HIV infection is an absolute contraindication to routine marrow donation; conversely, donor seropositivity for hepatitis B or C is probably not an absolute contraindication, but will likely greatly complicate the procedure.

Patient Considerations

As noted by other authors (see reviews in the bibliography), the sequential phases of the marrow transplantation procedure are associated with varying deficiencies of the immune system. Therefore, different types of infections tend to occur at more-or-less specific times post-transplant.

Pre-Transplant Phase (Before Day 0)

Patients are heterogeneous in terms of their immune status pre-transplant. Leukemic patients in chemotherapy-induced early remission (or first stable phase) may have relatively normal immune function, whereas patients with more advanced leukemia, lymphoma, myeloma and (most obviously) those with immunodeficiency diseases may have significant immune impairment. Moreover, some patients, especially those who have been extensively treated, may have acquired specific infections or have had procedures or devices (such as indwelling central venous or right atrial lines) that may predispose to later problems with infection.

Of special concern are those patients with unresolved serious infections who require urgent transplants (e.g., an untransfused severe aplastic anemia patient); while such infections may be difficult or impossible to control after transplantation, the resolution of such infections may depend on the recovery from neutropenia (and/or other immune components) that will result only from a successful marrow transplant. In this case, appropriate anti-microbial therapy and the transplant must be given in close sequence, possibly concomitantly, albeit with the acceptance of increased short-term risk of morbidity and mortality.

Factors that may predispose the patient to infection post-transplant must be evaluated before the transplant sequence begins. Such factors include, but are not limited to, the presence and status of indwelling intravenous devices, the presence of organ obstruction with tumor masses (or more benign etiologies), and evidence of a previous infection (especially CMV and herpes simplex virus [HSV], but also tuberculosis, aspergillosis, etc.). Moreover, special consideration should be given to patients from certain endemic areas for infections unusual to the geographic area of the transplant center (e.g., *Strongyloides stercoralis*). As above, active infections require that prompt treatment be instituted, and ideally completed, before conditioning begins. In any except the most straightforward infections, consultation with an infectious disease specialist with experience in the infectious problems of marrow transplantation may be helpful.

It is unclear whether certain patients with a history of deep fungal infection that is difficult to eradicate should be excluded from subsequent transplantation; hepatosplenic candidiasis and pulmonary aspergillosis in acute leukemia patients who have undergone prior chemotherapy are perhaps the most common examples of this dilemma. Although both infections are very difficult to eradicate, neither is an absolute contraindication to later marrow transplantation. However, special measures will need to be taken in such patients – in addition to adequate treatment pre-transplant – perhaps including surgical resection of pulmonary aspergillosis and prolonged antifungal treatment post-transplant. Obviously, increased morbidity and mortality may be expected, and such patients should be selected very carefully.

Immediate Post-Transplant Phase (Day 0 to Day +30)

Due both to the profound neutropenia that is observed either at some time before or soon after completion of the conditioning regimen (including an absolute neutrophil count [ANC] less than $0.1 \times 10^9/L$ for several weeks) and to skin and mucosal disruption due to the effects of conditioning, infections caused by gram-positive and gram-negative bacteria as well as fungal organisms (usually *Candida sp.* or *Aspergillus sp.*) are frequent.

Bacteremia is often the most commonly identified infection; mucosal disruption is critical in the development of sepsis due to certain gram-negative aerobes (*Escherichia coli*, *Klebsiella pneumoniae* and *Pseudomonas aeruginosa*). Likewise, the presence of indwelling central venous catheters predisposes to gram-positive sepsis with skin organisms (coagulase-negative staphylococci, *Staphlococcus aureus* and streptococci). While most coagulase-negative staphylococci are of low virulence even in this setting, streptococcal infection often results in a fulminant course and fatal outcome.

Unfortunately, the clinical diagnosis of these infections is complicated both by confusion with the tissue damage resulting from conditioning and by the lack of many of the classical signs of inflammation due to severe neutropenia; although fever is common, it is non-specific and may also be due to medications or transfusions. In addition to the blood, the lungs are an especially common site of infection, and the perirectal area, skin, mouth and sinuses are also frequently involved. However, virtually any site may become infected, and assessment on a daily or twice-daily basis, with meticulous attention to the emergence or progression of subtle signs (e.g., perirectal tenderness) is important in the ongoing evaluation of such patients. (Conversely, it should be recognized that some features of a routine physical examination – notably digital rectal examination – should be avoided unless specifically indicated, as the possibility of inducing perirectal infection is felt to outweigh diagnostic advantages in the usual case.)

It is most important to remember that severe infection may occur in either localized or systemic forms without significant physical stigmata. Moreover, rapid diagnostic procedures are not generally reliable or universally available, further limiting precise and rapid diagnosis. The therapeutic implications of these factors are discussed below.

Prophylactic Measures

Given the frequency and the high morbidity (and occasional mortality) associated with infections during neutropenia, such infections should obviously be prevented if possible. Prophylaxis may be considered in three general categories: physical measures, chemoprophylaxis and immunoprophylaxis.

Good general hygenic measures (by both patient and staff), including meticulous handwashing, chlorhexidine mouthwashes, careful attention to the care of indwelling catheters, low-bacterial content food, avoidance of exposure to fresh flowers or plants, and high-efficiency particulate air (HEPA) filtration (primarily to prevent airborne spread of *Aspergillus sp.* infections) are important; masking and gowning is of doubtful benefit. In the broadest sense, the use of a "total protective environment" (including decontamination of the patient's skin and bowel flora, sterile food and laminar air flow [LAF]) as prophylaxis is effective in decreasing certain acquired infections but is very labor-intensive and therefore expensive, and has not uniformly improved survival. Relatively few centers use this approach exclusively.

Initial efforts regarding chemoprophylaxis were concentrated on the use of broad-spectrum non-resorbable antibiotics; although a reduction in infections was sometimes achieved, these drugs were of arguable overall benefit as compliance was poor, cost was high, and superinfections were frequent. More recent studies show that the selective depletion of aerobic bacteria with systemic antibiotics (especially co-trimoxazole and ciprofloxacin) may provide effective prophylaxis against certain gram-negative aerobes without excessive superinfection. However, it should be remembered that co-trimoxazole is inactive against *Pseudomonas sp.* and may produce additional myelosuppression, and that some centers are reporting cases of ciprofloxacin resistance in the case of prolonged neutropenia; this important issue is not resolved.

Since the most frequent fungal organisms are acquired in different ways (i.e., *Candida sp.* via the gastrointestinal tract and *Aspergillus sp.* from the air), the modes of prophylaxis for these organisms vary. Suppression of *Candida sp.* is somewhat controversial, although most investigators do not believe the use of oral nystatin or oral amphotericin B is very effective. There are also problems with 5-flucytosine (bone marrow suppression) and ketoconazole (interaction with cyclosporine); data with miconazole are equivocal, but it is also probably not very effective. More recently, fluconazole has been utilized, but is not clearly of proven benefit, and episodes of *C. kruseii* and *Torlopusus sp.* superinfection have been noted. Itraconazole should be evaluated, and is of more interest as it has much more activity against *Aspergillus sp.* than fluconazole. Somewhat surprisingly, the use of relatively low doses of amphotericin B (e.g., 0.1–0.2 mg/day, beginning on day +1 and continuing throughout hospitalization) may be effective and not very toxic. Nevertheless, such therapy is also not yet standard.

As noted above, HEPA-filtration is important in preventing or diminishing airborne fungal infections; however, some facilities have more problems with *Aspergillus sp.* infections than others, and HEPA-filtration may not be an absolute requirement in the latter. In the absence of HEPA-filtration, an alternative may be the use of nebulized amphotericin B (or perhaps oral or intravenous itraconazole); conversely, amphotericin B nasal spray is not of clear benefit.

Prophylactic or suppressive therapy for certain viral infections is also very important. The reactivation of HSV I/II occurs commonly in the immediate post-transplant period but only in seropositive patients; these infections can be confused with therapy-induced mucositis and may cause considerable morbidity. Suppressive doses of acyclovir (e.g., 125–250 mg/m^2 iv q 6–8h day −5 to +30) are effective and strongly recommended. Rarely, HSV resistance to acyclovir occurs and alternative antiviral therapy with foscarnet should be considered.

Recent observations indicate that the use of various immunoglobulin preparations or ganciclovir may prevent severe CMV infections in seropositive donor-patient pairs. Similar data exist for high-dose acyclovir (i.e., 500 mg/m^2 q 8 hours), but since acyclovir is less effective (and more expensive), its use in this manner is not recommended. It is likely that the use of ganciclovir will become widespread in CMV-seropositive donor-recipient pairs, although it is not entirely clear whether such should be limited to particular high-risk groups (e.g., those patients receiving glucocorticoids and/or those with GVHD) or to all seropositive patients. Foscarnet will also be evaluated in this role.

Regarding immunoprophylaxis, certain immunoglobulin preparations have been shown to reduce bacterial infection in the allogeneic but less clearly in the autologous marrow transplant situation, a finding that may be related to the reduction in acute GVHD noted in some immunoglobulin prophylaxis studies. In any case, immunoglobulin therapy is costly and is not routinely indicated for infection prophylaxis alone – simpler and less expensive modalities exist. Similarly, prophylactic neutrophil transfusions are not indicated due to their marginal efficacy, the risk of allosensitization, the potential for transmission of various infections (especially CMV), the emergence of resistant organisms, and potential pulmonary toxicity.

Clearly, the use of hematopoietic growth factors to shorten the period of neutropenia (and ideally, pancytopenia) will be a major factor in reducing certain of these infections. As of this writing, it appears that the use of granulocyte colony-stimulating factor (G-CSF) or granulocyte-macrophage colony-stimulating factor (GM-CSF) is now standard therapy in autologous transplants for lymphoproliferative and certain non-hematologic malignancies. This is not yet the case for allogeneic transplants, perhaps due to the use of the myelosuppressive agent methotrexate in GVHD prophylaxis, and in transplants of any kind for myeloid malignancy in many patients, in which the potential to augment residual clonogenic tumor exists. Nevertheless, there is no reason to assume that the use of other factors (or different schedules of G- or GM-CSF) will not be effective in allogeneic transplants as well. This would be especially desirable in situations in which delayed engraftment is anticipated (e.g., T-cell depletion, histoincompatibility – and especially both), although it is unrealistic to suppose that current growth factors will reverse marrow graft rejection per se. In any case, the potential impact of these agents is profound, and it is likely that the use of G- and GM-CSF, probably combined with other growth factors, will become routine in many other marrow transplant situations within the next few years.

Therapeutic Measures

Inadequately-treated infection can be rapidly fatal in the immediate post-transplant setting. Because profound neutropenia minimizes the typical signs of infection and rapid confirmatory laboratory tests to aid in diagnosis are not widely available, febrile (i.e., >38°C) neutropenic patients (especially those with an ANC < 0.5×10^9/L) should be given immediate empiric broad-spectrum antimicrobial therapy. This recommendation applies to virtually all such patients – even those with other potential causes of fever such as transfusions, since these do not preclude the possibility of infection. If the fever is confirmed to be of non-infectious origin, antibiotics can be stopped after a few doses, although one should be quite confident of the etiology in such cases – a rare circumstance.

Of course, a full diagnostic evaluation (including an examination of the oral cavity, the indwelling intravenous catheter site and the perirectal area) is indicated, directing diagnostic methods to sites with subtle signs. Blood cultures before commencement of antibiotics are mandatory and should be repeated if no diagnosis is obtained and fever persists. Routine radiographs of the chest and facial sinuses may be helpful in some cases, although it should be stressed that the vast majority of these studies will be negative at the time of initial fever, and that their "cost-effectiveness" is unproven.

While the specifics of empiric therapy are controversial, an antipseudomonal penicillin (e.g., ticarcillin, mezlocillin or piperacillin) and an aminoglycoside (e.g., gentamicin, tobramycin, amikacin) in combination are often used; the effective use of the latter requires periodic serum assays. Antibiotic combinations (e.g., two β-lactams such as ceftazidime and piperacillin) have been used with similar efficacy, and there is no clearly "optimal" regimen. An interesting approach is the use of antibiotic monotherapy with agents such as ceftazidime, imipenem or ciproflaxacin, as such is attractive from the standpoint of toxicity (and resultant cost-reduction); however, monotherapy with these agents is not yet standard practice, and may be best reserved for the stable patient with an ANC between $0.5-1.0 \times 10^9$/L. Of course, the choice of a specific empiric antibiotic regimen should be based, at least to a degree, upon the patterns of infection in one's own institution, and of course modified if a discrete organism is identified.

Routine gram-positive coverage is also somewhat controversial, to some degree due to the cost (and to a lesser degree, toxicity) of vancomycin, the drug of choice. While vancomycin is needed to prevent the serious complications that often attend *S. viridans* or *S. aureus sepsis*, *S. epidermidis* infections associated with the use of indwelling intravenous catheters are of relatively low virulence, even in the transplant setting, and some workers have argued that this expensive treament should be delayed until evidence of such is documented. Conversely, and in order to minimize the potentially serious sequelae of the more virulent organisms, vancomycin may be given empirically for approximately 72 hours after the occurrence of fever; its use is then reassessed after a culture results are available, and discontinued unless a specific reason for its continuation – especially a positive culture of a sensitive organism – is present. However, even when a positive culture for the gram-positive organism is obtained, broad-spectrum antibiotics directed against gram-negative organisms should be given while neutropenia persists. A new agent, teicoplanin, may be an attractive alternative to vancomycin due to its reduced nephrotoxicity and use of a once-daily schedule.

For patients who respond to antibiotics, therapy is usually continued for at least 5–7 days, and ideally until after the ANC exceeds $0.5 \times 10^9/L$. Although in stable patients the discontinuance of this therapy may be considered even if the ANC is less than $0.5 \times 10^9/L$, patients with moderate or severe acute GVHD should be continued on antibiotics at least until the GVHD is under control.

Conversely, for patients persistently febrile after 3–7 days of antimicrobial therapy, and especially those who develop recurrent fever after an initial response to antibiotics but show no additional evidence of infection, recommendations are more variable. Although non-infectious causes of fever must of course be excluded, it is nonetheless generally assumed that infection is not controlled in this situation, and a full re-evaluation (including sinus and chest radiographs) is required; invasive studies may also be indicated, especially if a possible site of infection is found. The presence of diagnostic cultures, however, does not guarantee that the same organism involves all sites. This is especially the case in patients with prolonged neutropenia who develop bacteremia and lung infiltrates; the latter may be due to fungal organisms. In any case, failure to demonstrate a specific organism or site is not adequate justification for discontinuing all antimicrobial therapy.

To some degree, the next therapeutic step, if empiric, would depend on the primary therapy. For instance, if vancomycin has been utilized previously, it may be added; if monotherapy with imipenem has been used, an aminoglycoside may be added. However, the major question that arises in this situation regards the addition of antifungal treatment with amphotericin B, the only proven antifungal agent in this setting. This decision will usually need to be made on an empiric basis, as the deep fungal infections that are common in this circumstance (especially in patients with prolonged neutropenia) are very difficult to diagnose antemortem and are highly lethal; they must be treated early and vigorously. Unfortunately, amphotericin B is nephrotoxic, and the concomitant use of cyclosporine or aminoglycosides often worsens this problem. Alternative preparations (e.g., liposomal amphotericin B) or various agents designed to reduce the toxicity of amphotericin B on the kidney (e.g., "renal-dose" dopamine or pentoxifylline [see IV.7]) may be useful but are not yet considered standard.

As noted above, since amphotericin B is the only proven therapy in this serious situation, it should not be used timidly; daily doses of 0.5–1.0 mg/kg/day are usually required, treating to cumulative doses of >1 g (and occasionally >3 g). The dose of amphotericin B may need to be altered to minimize nephrotoxicity if this is a significant problem. One may reduce or delete other medications that may also cause (or augment) nephrotoxicity, if at all possible; this statement applies more to aminoglycosides rather than cyclosporine. Finally, preliminary evidence suggests that macrophage-colony stimulating factor (M-CSF) may be useful for resistant fungal infections, but such use is investigational.

Additional strategies regarding the treatment of persistent or recurrent fever include removal of indwelling intravenous catheters, which should always be considered as a potential source of infection or fever. However, their removal – even in the presence of infection – is usually not necessary unless one of the following is observed: 1) persistent sepsis despite appropriate antimicrobial coverage; 2) tunnel infection; 3) fungemia; or 4) clot at the catheter tip in the presence of sepsis. Identification of certain bacterial organisms (e.g., *Bacillus sp.* and *Corynebacterium JK*) may also be indications for removal of the catheter. (It should also be removed if a non-infected thrombus is identified.) In any event, these intravenous lines must be meticulously cared for by trained personnel – including the patient and family after discharge. Other imaging studies and leukocyte scans may be helpful in individual cases. Nevertheless, negative results of such an evaluation should not be used to delay the routine use of empiric therapy.

Infectious diarrhea is another problem during this time, and may be augmented by (or confused with) effects of the conditioning regimen, prolonged systemic or non-resorbable antibiotics, or other medications or GVHD. While a variety of organisms may cause this diarrhea, it is important to obtain stool cultures and assays for *Clostridium difficile* toxin in all except the most transient diarrheas; treatment with oral metronidozole or vancomycin is indicated. Moreover, certain other bacterial, viral or protozoal etiologies of diarrhea may be present; such should be fully investigated, and treated if possible.

Post-transplant viral infection of the liver is discussed in III.6, and of the bladder in III.7.

Other Measures

Therapeutic neutrophil transfusions are also seldom used at present due to their limited efficacy and potential toxicity. However, they may occasionally be considered for highly-selected patients who have clear evidence of infection (usually gram-negative sepsis) with a suboptimal early response to conventional antibiotics and who are at risk for prolonged neutropenia – or when the infecting organisms appear resistant to tested antibiotics. Since the lack of efficacy of neutrophil transfusions may be related to the relatively low number of cells transfused in some cases, the use of more than a single transfusion per day may be of greater benefit in desperate situations. Anti-endotoxin monoclonal antibodies are being evaluated for the treatment of septic shock in non-transplanted patients, and may prove useful in the marrow transplant setting as well.

The treatment of presumed or putative neutropenic infection with available hematopoietic growth factors has not been fully evaluated; although one would anticipate that this approach might be very cost-effective if limited to those patients actually infected, in whom routine antimicrobials were less useful, the roughly 1-week delay in producing neutrophils that is associated with the use of G- or GM-CSF could be problematic. Nevertheless, such should be considered in selected cases. Moreover, it is at least arguable that an ANC of $> 1.5 \times 10^9$/L may be more helpful than lesser levels in some cases.

Also, hematopoietic growth factors are potentially very useful in the setting of graft failure, and are probably indicated – despite the equivocal results noted to date with GM-CSF in this situation; combinations of (as yet) unavailable growth factors will likely be more effective. Due to the high mortality of graft failure, the potential adverse effects (including an increased rate of relapse in the myeloid malignancies) should not be considered a reason to avoid these agents in this situation.

Intermediate Post-Transplant Phase (Day +30 to +100)

After ANC recovery to $> 0.5 \times 10^9$/L, which generally occurs before day +30 in uncomplicated situations, the bacterial and fungal infections discussed above usually improve. However, they may not always resolve – particularly in the presence of GVHD, which can be associated with additional defects of neutrophil function.

If moderate-to-severe acute GVHD occurs, its treatment requires additional immunosuppressive therapy. Accordingly, most of the serious infections seen during this phase are in patients with GVHD. Whether GVHD is always primary in this circumstance is unclear, as infection-reducing total protective environment facilities have been shown to reduce acute GVHD in some transplanted patients. (This finding may be analogous to the decreased incidence of GVHD in gnotobiotic animals, and gives added impetus to infection prevention.) In any case that prompt and successful therapy (or, ideally, prevention) of GVHD will reduce such infections; the converse may be true as well.

A frequent site of infections during this period is the lung; this may be related to certain elements of conditioning regimens (especially total body irradiation) and a general impairment of mucociliary action. Such lung infections may be focal, and if so are often due to bacteria or fungi. Frequently, however, a diffuse interstitial pattern is noted radiographically; these are generally referred to as "interstitial pneumonias" and are often due to viral agents, notably CMV, although cases of HSV, adenovirus and respiratory syncytial virus interstitial pneumonitis have also been reported. (In many cases, no specific agent is identified, even with direct tissue examination; these cases are referred to as "idiopathic".) Other non-infectious pulmonary complications such as pulmonary edema, alveolar hemorrhage, transfusion-associated infiltrates, disease recurrence and – most arguably – involvement of the lung by GVHD should be considered; invasive diagnostic techniques are almost always required. Regardless of the specific agent or etiology, the mortality of this process is high. (The etiology, prevention and treatment of interstitial pneumonias are discussed more fully in III.5.)

Fortunately, effective prophylaxis may be administered to prevent CMV-interstitial pneumonitis in some circumstances – specifically, the use of CMV-negative blood products in CMV-seronegative donor-patient pairs or, less clearly, of intravenous immunoglobulin with a high CMV titer. The role of these measures in seropositive pairs is speculative, and given the high cost of immunoglobulin preparations, neither is clearly indicated in those patients (although it is certainly reasonable to consider the goal of "virus-negative" blood to be worthwhile for all transplant patients). Recently, the use of ganciclovir has been shown to be effective in preventing CMV-interstitial pneumonitis in seropositive patients with asymptomatic viremia or positive cultures in broncho-alveolar lavage specimens at roughly 5 weeks post-transplant. Also, routine use of ganciclovir for several weeks after marrow engraftment has preliminarily reduced the incidence of CMV infections in seropositive patients, although blood count suppression may be of concern. Foscarnet is potentially useful in this situation by virtue of its different spectrum of toxicity, but has been much less well studied.

Another major infectious cause of interstitial pneumonitis is *Pneumocystis carinii*. Fortunately, relatively low doses of trimethoprim-sulfamethoxazole (e.g., one double-strength tablet bid on weekends or thrice weekly) is effective prophylaxis in almost all patients. Patients with true intolerance to trimethoprim-sulfamethoxazole can receive nebulized (inhaled) or intravenous pentamidine, although much less data (and some doubt) exist regarding equivalent efficacy to trimethoprim-sulfamethoxazole.

While the management of patients with interstitial pneumonitis is controversial, an aggressive approach to obtaining tissue is usually recommended. Ideally, bronchoscopy and bronchoalveolar lavage should be performed within the first few hours after presentation. Special rapid-diagnostic techniques (especially those for CMV, *Legionella pneumophilia* and *Pneumocystis carinii*) should be performed. If these assays are non-diagnostic or not helpful, an open lung biopsy should be arranged promptly; even in a precariously ill patient, this can usually be performed safely by a skilled surgical team with meticulous attention to hemostasis.

Although not routinely recommended, an alternative approach to invasive techniques is to use broad-spectrum empiric therapy, covering the usual organisms involved. Although the morbidity of the diagnostic procedure is avoided (at least initially) with this approach, the delay in instituting proper therapy (if such was not selected on an empirical basis) may be very deleterious. Also, there are many organisms that must be considered, and if the initial response is unsatisfactory further empiric agents or a subsequent invasive diagnostic procedure in a weakened patient will be required. Finally, an increase in adverse drug interactions and toxicity can be anticipated with this approach.

Specific therapies include ganciclovir and hyperimmune globulin for CMV, trimethoprim-sulfamethoxazole or intravenous pentamidine for *Pneumocystis carinii* and erythromycin for *Legionella pneumophilia*. Extensive supportive care is also required, although the need for assisted ventilation portends a poor outcome regardles of etiology.

Other infections commonly noted during this period include sinusitis (due to either bacteria or fungi), cutaneous infection, or sepsis due to indwelling central venous catheter infections. Rarely, other parasitic organisms (such as *Toxoplasma gondii*) may be noted.

Late Post-Transplant Phase (After Day +100)

In general, patients who reach this point are at less risk of serious infection – unless they have ongoing GVHD. However, many other patients remain immunosuppressed to some degree and are therefore at risk for various infectious complications, chiefly but not exclusively with bacterial and viral organisms.

The management of infections in the setting of chronic GVHD is an extremely important area, and is discussed in detail in IV.2. Local or disseminated bacterial infections (especially with encapsulated organisms such as *Streptococcus pneumoniae* and *Hemophilus influenzae*) are common; hyposplenism and specific IgG_2 subclass deficiency may be contributory. Prophylactic oral antibiotic coverage (e.g., using trimethoprim-sulfamethoxazole, or alternatively, in intolerant patients, penicillin) has been found effective and is strongly recommended. The role of immunoprophylaxis is not fully defined but such may be helpful in selected patients. Unfortunately, routine immunization is usually not useful in patients with chronic GVHD, primarily due to poor antibody response.

Conversely, routine re-immunization is required in patients without chronic GVHD at about 1 year post-transplant. The general rule is to exclude live attenuated viral vaccines, although these have been given in some cases without obvious problems. One recommendation is to give the diphtheria/ tetanus (DT) vaccine and assess response 6–8 weeks later by measuring tetanus toxoid antibody levels. If a response is noted, pneumoccocal vaccine, meningococcal vaccine and *Hemophilus influenza* (HIB) protein conjugate vaccine should be administered. Booster vaccine for the pneumoccocal, meningococcal and HIB is advised at about 24 months posttransplant. Killed polio (Salk) vaccine should be given 1–2 years after transplant. Contacts of transplant patients should not receive oral live polio vaccine, but may receive measles/mumps/rubella (MMR) vaccine.

Certain viral infections are also noted during this time. Although CMV-interstitial pneumonitis is uncommon, it is almost always seen in the setting of chronic GVHD (see IV.2). More frequent are *varicella zoster* infections. Although zoster infections usually remain localized, they can disseminate, and are often associated with considerable morbidity and occasional mortality. Systemic acyclovir (10–12 mg/kg intravenously every 8 hours) is indicated for all cases of zoster with multidermatome or disseminated disease, and it may be considered for other patients as well. Since the mortality of these infections is relatively low, it would be desirable to avoid hospitalization; the use of high-dose oral acyclovir (i.e., 800 mg po × 5 per day) is an interesting alternative, albeit of unproven efficacy.

The development of the acquired immunodeficiency disease syndrome (AIDS) due to transmission of HIV via blood products is now a relatively rare problem in marrow transplant patients, due to improved screening of blood products. Patients and donors should be screened for HIV before transplantation, and patients should be checked again several months following transplantation. Infection with HIV should also be considered when patients have unexplained opportunistic infections later in their treatment courses than would otherwise be expected, especially in the absence of GVHD.

As detailed in IV.6, there is some evidence that the Epstein-Barr virus (EBV) drives the development of certain complicating B-cell cancers, especially in patients with severe and prolonged GVHD. As with other transplant-related malignancies, immunosuppression should be discontinued if possible; α-interferon and/or acyclovir may be useful.

Future Directions

Since many of the most serious infectious complications after bone marrow transplantation are found in patients with severe neutropenia (especially if prolonged by graft failure) and those with severe GVHD, control of these problems would greatly decrease the morbidity and mortality associated with infection. The use of recombinant growth factors to shorten the period of immunosuppression will undoubtedly be explored extensively within the next few years, and potentially holds great promise. Also, the ability to specifically augment the post-transplant immune system with certain cytokines is an exciting goal.

Regardless of these efforts, however, the development of improved antimicrobial agents – especially agents with more activity against fungal and viral organisms, and ideally ones capable of being given by the oral route – would also be most helpful.

References

Anaissie E, Bodey GP, Kantarjian H, Ro J, Vartivarian SE, Hopfer R, Hoy J, Rolston K (1989) New spectrum of fungal infections in patients with cancer. Rev Infect Dis 11:369

Barnes RA, Rogers TRF (1989) Control of an outbreak of nosocomial aspergillosis by laminar air-flow isolation. J Hosp Infect 14:89

Benhamou E, Hartmann O, Nogues C, Maraninchi D, Valteau D, Lemerle J (1991) Does ketoconazole prevent fungal infection in children treated with high dose chemotherapy and bone marrow transplantation? Results of a randomized placebo-controlled trial. Bone Marrow Transplant 7:127

Bowden RA, Sayers M, Flournoy N, Newton B, Banaji M, Thomas ED, Meyers JD (1986) Cytomegalovirus immune globulin and seronegative blood products to prevent primary cytomegalovirus infection after marrow transplantation. N Engl J Med 314:1006

Chan CK, Hyland RH, Hutcheon MA (1990) Pulmonary complications following bone marrow transplantation. Clin Chest Med 11:323

Conneally E, Cafferkey MT, Daly PA, Keane CT, McCann SR (1990) Nebulized amphotericin B as prophylaxis against invasive aspergillosis in granulocyopenic patients. Bone Marrow Transplant 5:403

De Pauw BE, Donnelly JP, De Witte T, Novakova IRO, Schattenberg A (1990) Options and limitations of long-term oral ciprofloxacin as antibacterial prophylaxis in allogeneic bone marrow transplant recipients. Bone Marrow Transplant 5:179

Ferretti GA, Ash RC, Brown AT, Parr MD, Romond EH, Lillich TT (1988) Control of oral mucositis and candidiasis in marrow transplantation: A prospective, double-blind trial of chlorhexidine digluconate oral rinse. Bone Marrow Transplant 3:483

Hughes WT, Armstrong D, Bodey GP, Feld R, Mandell GL, Meyers JD, Pizzo PA, Schimpff SC, Shenep JL, Wade JC, Young LS, Yow MD (1990) Guidelines for the use of antimicrobial agents in neutropenic patients with unexplained fever. J Infect Dis 161:381

Karp JE, Merz WG, Dick JD, Saral R (1991) Strategies to prevent or control infections after bone marrow transplants. Bone Marrow Transplant 8:1

Kureishi A, Jewesson PJ, Rubinger M, Cole CD, Reece DE, Phillips GL, Smith JA, Chow AW (1991) Double-blind comparison of teicoplanin versus vancomycin in febrile neutropenic patients receiving concomitant tobramycin and piperacillin: Effect on cyclosporin A-associated nephrotoxicity. Antimicrob Agents Chemother 35:2246

Lum LG (1987) The kinetics of immune reconstitution after human marrow transplantation. Blood 69:369

Nemunaitis J, Rabinowe SN, Singer JW, Bierman PJ, Vose JM, Freedman AS, Onetto N, Gillis S, Oette D, Gold M, Buckner CD, Hansen JA, Ritz J, Appelbaum FR, Armitage JO, Nadler LM (1991) Recombinant granulocyte-macrophage colony-stimulating factor after autologous bone marrow transplantation for lymphoid cancer. N Engl J Med 324:1773

Nemunaitis J, Singer JW, Buckner CD, Durnam D, Epstein C, Hill R, Storb R, Thomas ED, Appelbaum FR (1990) Use of recombinant human granulocyte-macrophage colony-stimulating factor in graft failure after bone marrow transplantation. Blood 76:245

O'Donnell MR, Schmidt GM, Tegtmeier B, Faucett C, Nademanee A, Parker PM, Smith EP, Snyder DS, Stein AS, Blume KG, Forman SJ (1990) Prophylactic low dose amphotericin B (AM-B) decreases systemic fungal infection (SFI) in allogeneic bone marrow transplant (BMT) recipients. Blood 76 Suppl 1:558a

Petersen FB, Clift RA, Hickman RO, Sanders JE, Meyers JD, Kelleher J, Buckner CD (1986) Hickman catheter complications in marrow transplant recipients. J Parenter Enter Nutr 10:58

Powles R, Smith C, Milan S, Treleaven J, Millar J, McElwain T, Gordon-Smith E, Milliken S, Tiley C (1990) Human recombinant GM-CSF in allogeneic bone-marrow transplantation for leukaemia: Double-blind, placebo-controlled trial. Lancet 336:1417

Reed EC, Myerson D, Corey L, Meyers JD (1991) Allogeneic marrow transplantation in patients positive for hepatitis B surface antigen. Blood 77:195

Rogers TR (1991) Prevention of infection during neutropenia. Br J Haematol 79:544

Russell JA, Poon M-C, Jones AR, Woodman RC, Ruether BA (1992) Allogeneic bone-marrow transplantation without protective isolation in adults with malignant disease. Lancet 339:38

Shearer WT, Ritz J, Finegold MJ, et al. (1985) Epstein-Barr virus-associated B-cell proliferations of diverse clonal origins after bone marrow transplantation in a 12-year-old patient with severe combined immunodeficiency. N Engl J Med 312:1151

Storb R, Prentice RL, Buckner CD, Clift RA, Appelbaum F, Deeg J, Doney K, Hansen JA, Mason M, Sanders JE, Singer J, Sullivan KIM, Witherspoon RP, Thomas ED (1983) Graft-versus-host disease and survival in patients with aplastic anemia treated by marrow grafts from HLA-identical siblings: Beneficial effects of a protective environment. N Engl J Med 308:302

Sullivan KM, Kopecky KJ, Jocom J, Fisher L, Buckner CD, Meyers JD, Counts GW, Bowden RA, Petersen FB, Witherspoon RP, Budinger MD, Schwartz RS, Appelbaum FR, Clift RA, Hansen JA, Sanders JE, Thomas ED, Storb R (1990) Immunomodulatory and antimicrobial efficacy of intravenous immunoglobulin in bone marrow transplantation. N Engl J Med 323:705

Valteau D, Hartmann O, Brugieres L, Vassal G, Benhamou E, Andremont A, Kalifa C, Lemerle J (1991) Streptococcal septicaemia following autologous bone marrow transplantation in children treated with high-dose chemotherapy. Bone Marrow Transplant 7:415

Verfaillie C, Weisdorf R, Haake R, Hostetter M, Ramsay NKC, McGlave P (1991) Candida infections in bone marrow transplant recipients. Bone Marrow Transplant 8:177

Wingard JR (1990) Advances in the management of infectious complications after bone marrow transplantation. Bone Marrow Transplant 6:371

Wingard JR (1990) Management of infectious complications of bone marrow transplantation. Oncology (Williston Park) 4 (Feb):69

Winston DJ, Ho WG, Bruckner DA, Champlin RE (1991) Beta-lactam antibiotic therapy in febrile granulocytopenic patients: A randomized trial comparing cefoperazone plus piperacillin, ceftazidime plus piperacillin, and imipenem alone. Ann Intern Med 115:849

5. Interstitial Pneumonitis

Definition

Interstitial pneumonitis is usually of nonbacterial, nonfungal etiology. The disease process involves mostly the pulmonary interstitium in the form of mononuclear cell infiltration and fluid accumulation with a relative sparing of air spaces. The most common symptom is shortness of breath. Cough is nonproductive, unless a bacterial superinfection is present. The diagnosis is usually made by chest radiography along with blood gas analysis. Bronchoalveolar lavage is often, but not always, helpful in establishing the etiology (e.g., cytomegalovirus [CMV], P. carinii). Occasionally, a definitive diagnosis requires an open lung biopsy.

Etiology

Several etiological factors for the development of interstitial pneumonitis have been recognized (Table 20). An important cause is CMV which used to account for almost half the cases of interstitial pneumonitis observed after marrow transplantation. In a proportion of patients no infectious agent can be identified and these cases are referred to as "idiopathic." Clinical observations indicate, however, that idiopathic pneumonitis is at least in part related to irradiation, and in some instances possibly to chemotherapy. In earlier studies Pneumocystis carinii was found in 10–15% of cases; the introduction of trimethoprim/sulfamethoxazole prophylaxis has almost completely eliminated this disease. All other causes listed are infrequent.

Table 20. Etiology of interstitial pneumonitis

1. Infections
   - Viruses
   Pneumocystis carinii
   - Legionella
   - Chlamydia trachomatis
   - Cytomegalovirus (CMV)
   - Herpes simplex virus (HSV)
   - Adenovirus
   - Respiratory syncytial virus
   - Measles virus
   - Others
2. Irradiation
3. Chemical Causes
   - Cyclophosphamide
   - Busulfan
   - Carmustine
   - Methotrexate
4. Idiopathic

Table 21. Risk factors for the development of interstitial pneumonitis after marrow transplantation

- Allogeneic transplant
- Graft-vs-host disease
- Total body irradiation (TBI) for conditioning
- Higher exposure rate used for TBI
- Single dose TBI
- Prior radiotherapy to the chest
- Seropositivity for cytomegalovirus (CMV)
- Transfusion of CMV positive blood products
- Increasing patient age
- Methotrexate post-transplant
- Female donor sex
- Omission of trimethoprim/sulfamethoxazole prophylaxis

Risk Factors and Epidemiology

Risk factors are listed in Table 21. Interstitial pneumonitis can occur one week or two years after transplantation; the peak incidence is at approximately 8–10 weeks. Idiopathic interstitial pneumonitis tends to occur earlier than CMV related pneumonitis. Recognized risk factors differ for cases of interstitial pneumonitis due to different etiologies.

Patients given an allogeneic transplant have a significantly higher probability of developing CMV pneumonitis than patients given a syngeneic or autologous transplant. In fact, in the first 100 patients given a syngeneic transplant in Seattle, no case of CMV pneumonitis was identified. In agreement with the concept that allogenecity contributes to the development of CMV pneumonitis is the observation that this entity increases in frequency with the severity of GVHD in the recipient. No such correlation has been recognized for idiopathic interstitial pneumonitis, which appears to occur with similar frequency in patients given allogeneic, syngeneic or autologous transplants, and in patients with and without GVHD.

Patients transplanted for severe aplastic anemia have a lower incidence of interstitial pneumonitis than patients transplanted for lymphohemopoietic malignancies. Although it is conceivable that the underlying diagnosis itself or treatment given before transplantation represent risk factors, it is clear that the conditioning used in preparation for transplantation is of importance. Until recently most patients with lymphohemopoietic malignancies were conditioned with regimens including the use of TBI. Most patients with non-malignant disorders including severe aplastic anemia have been conditioned with chemotherapy only or, if TBI was used, generally at lower total doses than in patients with lymphohemopoietic malignancies.

Over the past decade the incidence of interstitial pneumonitis has declined. A major factor has been the use of fractionated rather than single-dose TBI. It was of note that TBI dose fractionation had its major impact on idiopathic interstitial pneumonitis, and much less on the incidence of CMV pneumonitis. The beneficial effect of fractionated TBI on idiopathic interstitial pneumonitis was most prominent in patients given methotrexate rather than cyclosporine as GVHD prophylaxis. There is also evidence that patients with a diagnosis of Hodgkin disease or non-Hodgkin lymphoma, who received irradiation to the chest or the mediastinum before coming to marrow transplantation have a significantly higher probability of developing idiopathic interstitial pneumonitis than patients without prior radiotherapy. This notion is supported by the results of a recent analysis of patients with prior chest radiotherapy showing an incidence of interstitial pneumonitis of 30–35% if conditioned with TBI, compared to 5–10% when conditioned with chemotherapy only. Furthermore, a recent analysis by the International Bone Marrow Transplantation Registry suggests that patients given TBI at an exposure rate of ≥5.7 cGy/min have a higher incidence of pneumonitis than patients irradiated at lower exposure rates.

The most significant risk factor for the development of CMV pneumonitis is the CMV immune status of patient and donor. The lowest incidence of CMV pneumonitis is observed in patients who have no evidence of prior exposure to CMV (CMV negative), and who are being transplanted from a similarly CMV negative donor. If the donor is positive for CMV, the risk of developing significant CMV infection even in a CMV negative recipient, is increased. If the patient is CMV positive, the risk increases substantially, and does not appear to be significantly affected by the donor CMV status. Consequently, the transfusion of CMV positive blood products also represents a risk factor for CMV pneumonitis, at least in patients who are CMV negative. As discussed below (Prophylaxis), the use of CMV-negative blood products, and leukocyte filters, the prophylactic use of acyclovir on the early "preemptive" treatment of CMV excretion with ganciclovir has substantially reduced the incidence of CMV disease.

Other risk factors that have been described such as patient age, female donor sex, the interval from diagnosis to transplant and the performance rating before transplantation are more controversial.

Pathogenesis

The presence of an infectious agent in the immunosuppressed patient will lead to an inflammatory reaction, presumably facilitated by a direct toxic effect of the conditioning regimen on pulmonary tissue. This inflammatory reaction involves mononuclear cell infiltration and fluid accumulation and leads to thickening of the interstitium. The contribution of cytokines (e.g., tumor necrosis factor) and prostaglandin derivatives to this process is still incompletely understood. As a consequence of septal thickening, the diffusing distance for oxygen from the air space (alveoli) to the capillaries in the interstitium increases, and arterial oxygen concentration in the blood decreases. The patient senses hypoxemia and feels short of breath. Early in the course, only partial arterial oxygen pressure will fall and as a consequence of increase respiratory effort, pCO_2 may be lower than normal. There may be a mild degree of respiratory alkalosis. As the patient tires, there may be a slowly increasing retention of CO_2 in addition to hypoxemia. Along with a hypoxemic metabolism this will result in a combined metabolic/respiratory acidosis. As the patient is being treated by increased oxygen intake (FiO_2) initially by mask, and subsequently often via endotracheal intubation, there may be secondary damage to the alveolar lining due to prolonged high oxygen exposure. The end result is a wet, heavy, and stiff lung incapable of performing its functions.

Clinical and Laboratory Features

The interstitial process leads to hypoxemia with air hunger and shortness of breath. Auscultation of the lung may be completely unrevealing; in fact the lungs may be suspiciously silent. There may be some nonspecific crackling sounds. A chest radiograph will generally show interstitial markings, either localized or diffused. These markings can involve the bases of the lungs, the peripheral areas, or can lead to a complete "white out" of both lung fields (Figs 5a,b and 6). Usually there will be fever but an occasional patient may be afebrile, which is not surprising since many patients are on immunosuppressive therapy including steroids. Although the clinical picture of interstitial pneumonitis is rather typical, a conclusion as to its etiology is often not possible.

Sputum is hardly ever available for examination. Bronchoalveolar lavage, in the hands of experienced pulmonologists and pathologists may yield diagnostic findings in the majority of CMV-related cases, but is less helpful with idiopathic pneumonitis. In these cases the most reliable diagnostic procedure is open lung biopsy. Although there is concern about hemorrhage during and following the procedure, usually adequate platelet support can be provided to prevent major

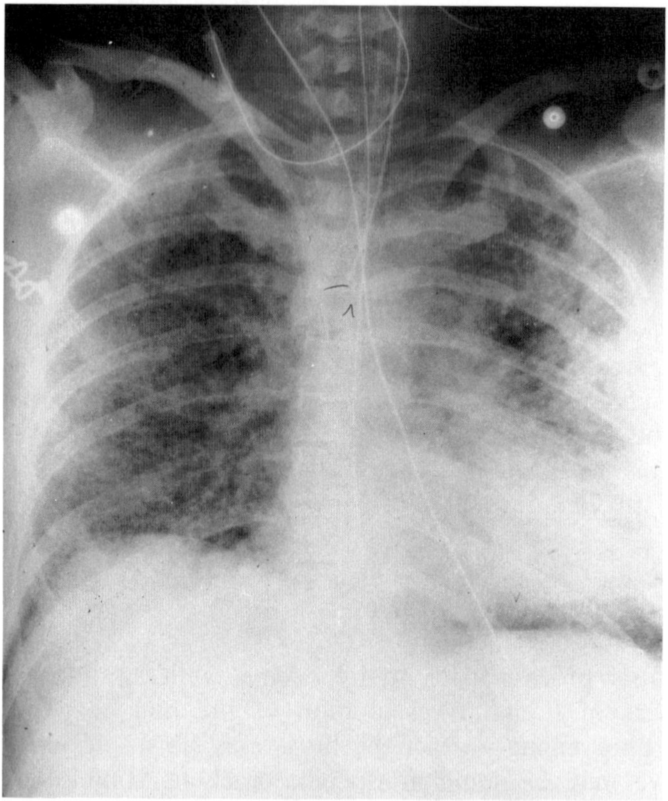
a

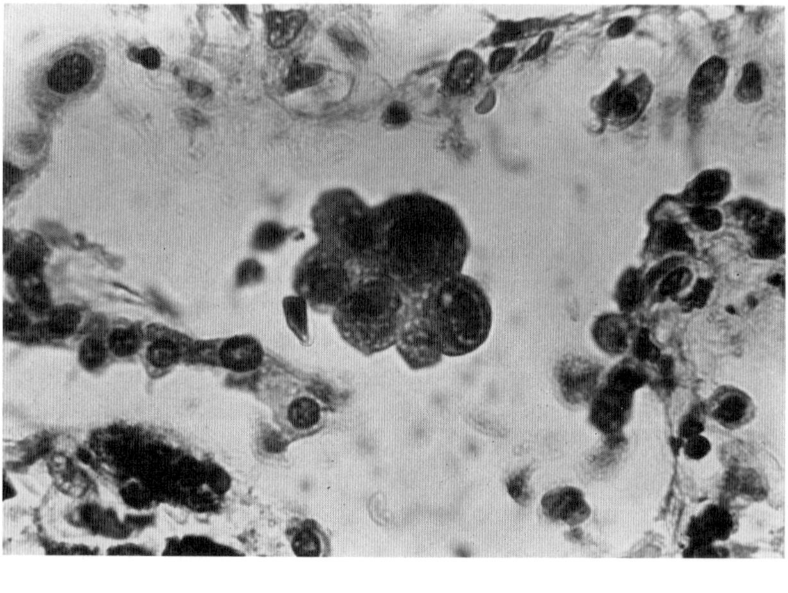
b

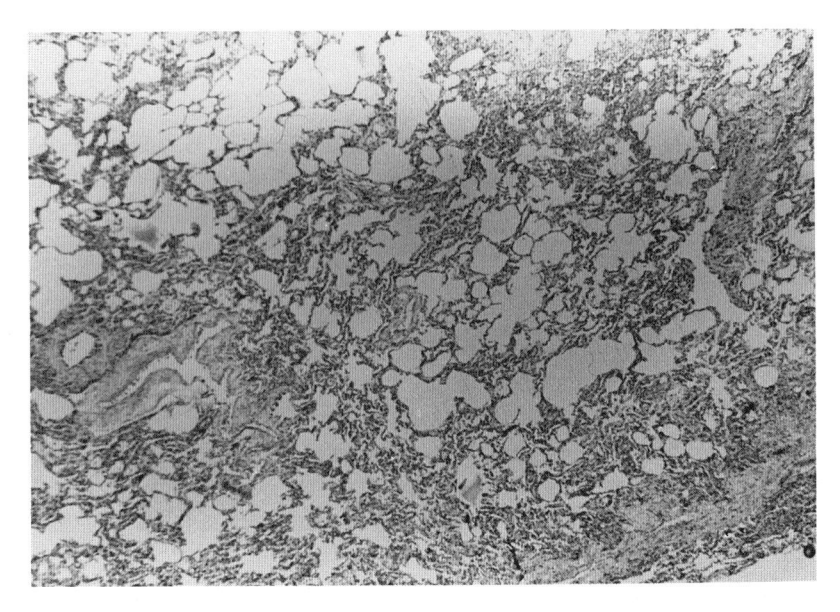

Fig. 6. Idiopathic interstitial pneumonitis showing thickened alveolar septa with edema and round cell infiltrates. No organisms identified

hemorrhages. Histological examination will reveal mononuclear cell infiltrates and fluid exudation into the interstitial space. There may be hemorrhage as well. In the case of CMV infection, characteristic intranuclear or cytoplasmatic inclusion bodies can be found (Figs 5a,b). In addition, virus may grow in culture. Concurrently, there may be an increase in the antibody titer against CMV as determined by complement fixation techniques or enzyme linked immunosorption assay. More recently monoclonal antibodies have become available that recognize certain protein structures of the virus which can be directly visualized by fluorescence techniques. As a research tool in situ hybridization with DNA probes complementary to certain CMV sequences can be utilized. Concurrently with the

←

Fig. 5a,b. Interstitial pneumonitis. Diffuse interstitial markings in both lung fields with a "white out" appearance in the left lower lobe (**a**). Tissue obtained at open lung biopsy reveals giant cells with cytoplasmatic and nuclear viral inclusion bodies characteristic of cytomegalovirus (**b**) development of pneumonitis, CMV may be present in the intestinal mucosa, throat or blood, or may be excreted in the urine.

Pneumocystis carinii pneumonitis is diagnosed when cysts of the organism are demonstrated in pulmonary tissue sections using stains such as silver methenamine or toluidine blue. In an occasional patient Pneumocystis can also be diagnosed from bronchial washings.

Herpes simplex virus, varicella zoster virus and adenovirus also cause inclusion bodies in cells of lung tissue. Some of them grow well in cultures causing characteristic cytopathic effects. Similar to the diagnosis of CMV pneumonitis, fluorescein labeled monoclonal antibodies specific for these viruses are now available for diagnostic purposes. Interstitial pneumonitis due to herpes virus frequently occurs in the setting of disseminated infection also involving the skin.

If complete examination of the tissue obtained at biopsy fails to reveal any organism, although the histological appearance is typical, usually the diagnosis of idiopathic interstitial pneumonitis is made (Fig. 6).

Differential Diagnosis

A patient presenting with shortness of breath, fever, and diffuse interstitial changes on chest radiograph is always suspected of having interstitial pneumonitis until proven otherwise. Fluid overload must be excluded as an etiology, particular if the picture develops early after transplantation, and in a setting of veno-occlusive disease of the liver or generalized capillary leak syndrome associated with a significant increase in body weight. In fact, veno-occlusive disease of pulmonary vessels has been described. An aggressive trial with diuretics provides a rapid answer; interstitial pneumonitis will not improve. Conceivably, a diffuse fungal pneumonia could resemble interstitial pneumonitis. This should be suspected when fungus, particularly Candida is grown from various culture sites including the sputum, but it may be necessary to obtain lung tissue to confirm the diagnosis. An acute respiratory distress syndrome associated with septicemia may resemble interstitial pneumonitis. Organisms such as Mycobacteria or Chlamydia may rarely cause pneumonitis, and the diagnosis will depend upon documentation of the organisms in tissue or the results of cultures.

Treatment and Prognosis

Historically, approximately 40% of all cases of interstitial pneumonitis were related to CMV. Agents such as vidarabine, interferon, and acyclovir have not significantly altered the disease course. The combined use of high-dose i.v. immunoglobulin (500 mg/kg every other day for two weeks) and ganciclovir results in disease resolution in 50% of patients. More effective is the prophylactic institution of ganciclovir in patients who excrete virus without showing clinical evidence of disease.

Pneumocystis carinii pneumonitis is treated with trimethoprim/sulfamethoxazole, which allows recovery in approximately 80–90% of patients. In patients with sulfa allergy, pentamidine can be used.

The rare cases of herpes simplex virus or varicella-zoster virus pneumonitis are treated most effectively with acyclovir.

No effective treatment is available for adenovirus. Respiratory syncytial virus is treated with vidarabin.

Mortality with idiopathic interstitial pneumonitis is in the range of 50–60%. Many investigators have used high-dose corticosteroids, and feel this is effective, although no controlled study has been performed.

Prevention

Since CMV has been the most frequent identifiable cause of interstitial pneumonitis many investigators have focused on this entity. The recognition that CMV is transmitted with leukocytes and the availability of acyclovir and ganciclovir have dramatically changed the impact of CMV post-transplant. In CMV negative patients transplanted from a CMV negative donor CMV infection and disease can be prevented virtually completely by using only CMV negative transfusion donors or by filtering all transfusion products. In CMV positive patients or in patients transplanted from a CMV positive donor, the prophylactic use of acyclovir beginning pre-transplant has significantly reduced CMV activation and disease. The institution of ganciclovir in those patients who begin to excrete virus further reduced the incidence of CMV disease. An additional reduction may be possible by instituting ganciclovir in all these patients once they have achieved engraftment ($\geq 0.75 \times 10^9$ granulocytes/L).

Pneumocystis carinii pneumonitis can be prevented by the prophylactic administration of trimethoprim/sulfamethoxazole beginning before transplantation and given for two days a week after transplantation for approximately 6 months in patients without GVHD; longer for patients with chronic GVHD (see below).

The incidence of idiopathic interstitial pneumonitis has decreased with the use of fractionated rather than single-dose TBI from approximately 13 to 5%. Whether cytokine inhibitors, e.g., pentoxifylline, can further improve these results is currently under investigation.

The development of acute GVHD increases the risk of CMV pneumonitis 2–3 times as compared to patients without GVHD. Consequently, every attempt must be made to reduce or prevent the development of GVHD. If GVHD develops and treatment is necessary, the use of antithymocyte globulin further increases the risk of CMV pneumonitis, and it might be advisable to use other agents such as steroids instead.

While the risk of interstitial pneumonitis in patients without chronic GVHD is limited to the first two to four months after transplantation, patients who develop extensive chronic GVHD may be at risk for several years. A recent study found late interstitial pneumonitis in 28 of 198 patients. It was idiopathic in 23%, due to CMV in 19%, due to pneumocystis carinii in 19%, and varicella zoster in 19%. Half of the patients died. The investigators showed that the probability of developing late interstitial pneumonitis was approximately 30% in patients who were not given antibiotic prophylaxis, but only

8% in patients who received prophylactic trimethoprim/sulfamethoxazole. The beneficial effect of this drug was mostly, although not exclusively, due to prevention of pneumocystis carinii pneumonitis.

These data clearly indicate that the prevention of both acute and chronic GVHD is desirable in order to prevent interstitial pneumonitis. Whether prolonged prophylactic administration of immunoglobulin preparations as currently investigated will prevent interstitial pneumonitis remains to be determined. It is also possible that late occurring pulmonary problems may be directly due to GVHD or associated infection. This has certainly been shown for obliterative bronchiolitis, and some interstitial processes responsive to immunosuppression have been described (see IV.3).

References

Barrett A, Depledge MH, Powles RL (1983) Interstitial pneumonitis following bone marrow transplantation after low dose rate total body irradiation. Int J Radiation Oncology Biol Phys 9:1029

Bowden RA, Sayers M, Flournoy N, Newton B, Banaji M, Thomas ED, Meyers JD (1986) Cytomegalovirus immune globulin and seronegative blood products to prevent primary cytomegalovirus infection after marrow transplantation. N Engl J Med 314:1006–1010

Bowden RA, Slichter SJ, Sayers MH, Mori M, Cays MJ, Meyers JD (1991) Use of leukocyte-depleted platelets and cytomegalovirus-seronegative red blood cells for prevention of primary cytomegalovirus infection after marrow transplant. Blood 78:246–250

Crawford SW (1991) The patient with leukemia and bone marrow transplantation. In: Tenholder MF (ed), Approach to Pulmonary Infection in the Immunocompromised Host. Futura Publishing Co, New York 167–206

Emanuel D, Cunningham I, Jules-Elysee K, Brochstein JA, Kerman NA, Laver J, Stover D, White DA, Fels A, Polsky B, Castro-Malaspina H, Peppard JR, Bartus P, Hammerling U, O'Reilly RJ (1988) Cytomegalovirus pneumonia after bone marrow transplantation successfully treated with the combination of ganciclovir and high-dose intravenous immune globulin. Ann Intern Med 109:777–782

Lonnqvist B, Ringden O, Wahren B, Gahrton G, Lundgren G (1984) Cytomegalovirus infection associated with and preceding chronic graft-versus-host disease. Transplantation 38:465–468

Meyers JD, Shepp DH, Bowden RA, Reed EC (1987) Viral infections in marrow transplant recipients. In: Gale RP, Champlin R (eds), Progress in Bone Marrow Transplantation, UCLA Symposia on Molecular and Cellular Biology, New Series, Vol. 53. Alan R. Liss, New York 545–562

Schmidt GM, Horak DA, Niland JC, Duncan SR, Forman SJ, Zaia JA (1991) A randomized, controlled trial of prophylactic ganciclovir for cytomegalovirus pulmonary infection in recipients of allogeneic bone marrow transplants. N Engl J Med 324:1005–1011

Shields AF, Hackman RC, Fife KH, Corey L, Meyers JD (1985) Adenovirus infections in patients undergoing bone marrow transplantation. N Engl J Med 312:529–533

Weiner RS, Bortin MM, Gale RP, Gluckman E, Kay HEM, Kolb H-J, Hartz AJ, Rimm AA (1986) Interstitial pneumonitis after bone marrow transplantation. Ann Intern Med 104:168–175

Wingard JR, Mellits ED, Sostrin MB, Chen DY-H, Burns WH, Santos GW, Vriesendorp HM, Beschorner WE, Saral R (1988) Interstitial pneumonitis after allogeneic bone marrow transplantation. Nine-year experience at a single institution. Medicine 67:175–186

Winston DJ, Ho WG, GAle RP, Champlin RE (1987) Treatment and prevention of interstitial pneumonia after bone marrow transplantation. In: Gale RP, Champlin (eds), Progress in Bone Marrow Transplantation. Alan R. Liss, New York 525

Zaia JA, Churchill MA (1987) The biology of human cytomegalovirus infection after marrow transplantation. In: Gale RP, Champlin R (eds), Progress in Bone Marrow Transplantation. Alan R. Liss, New York 563

6. Hepatic Dysfunction

Overview

Hepatic dysfunction frequently occurs after marrow transplantation. Time of onset, duration, treatment and prognosis are different for each clinical entity and the following etiologies must be distinguished:

– Veno-occlusive disease (VOD)
– Acute GVHD
– Chronic GVHD
– Infection
– Drug Injury
– Parenteral Nutrition
– Recurrent Malignancy

Veno-Occlusive Disease (VOD)

VOD is a consequence of toxic injury to the liver resulting from high-dose chemo- and radiotherapy used to condition the patient; it is the most common liver disease in the first months post-transplant and is clinically suspected if jaundice, weight gain and painful hepatomegaly develop in the first two weeks after marrow infusion. About 20–30% (and at some institutions up to 50%) of patients with malignancy prepared with a combination of chemotherapy or total body irradiation develop VOD. The incidence in patients undergoing autologous or syngeneic transplantation is lower, although the doses of chemo/radiotherapy are similar to those used for allogeneic transplantation. This led to speculation about a possible contribution of immunological mechanisms (i.e.,

GVHD) being involved in the pathogenesis of VOD although this has not been proven experimentally.

Pathogenesis

Active metabolites of antineoplastic agents may be concentrated in the pericentral (centrilobular) zone of the liver sinusoids, reaching toxic concentrations. The sinusoidal blood flow can then be obstructed by edematous, injured and necrotic hepatocytes, and, in addition, sinusoidal pores may be blocked by cellular debris and exfoliated hepatocytes. It is believed that release of tumor necrosis factor-alpha (TNF-α) potentiates cytotoxicity and activates coagulation leading to more severe obstruction of hepatic sinusoids and venules. This can cause a shift of fluid containing sodium and albumin from the intravascular to the extravascular space ("third space"). Since renal blood flow decreases, the kidneys react by activating the renin-angiotensin mechanism resulting in sodium retention. The clinical picture ultimately consists of peripheral fluid accumulation, hepatomegaly, abdominal pain, ascites, and impaired liver function with icterus. In severe cases with prolonged liver dysfunction, renal insufficiency may develop secondary to pre-renal failure and toxic tubular damage.

In patients treated with cyclosporine, an additional pathogenetic mechanism is thought to occur. Cyclosporine reduces prostacyclin release from endothelial cells, which may in turn cause coagulation abnormalities and facilitate capillary thrombosis. Such patients also have locally elevated levels of coagulation factor VIII and fibrinogen as well as increased aggregation of platelets. Therefore, cyclosporine-induced local coagulation abnormalities may be superimposed on chemo/radiotherapy related hepatic damage and contribute to the development of VOD.

Histopathology

Early changes include centrilobular congestion or hemorrhage (fragmented red cells), subendothelial edema, and fibrillar material. Intermediate changes are characterized by the occlusion of the venular lumina by collagen fibers (subendothelial), and atrophy of pericentral hepatocytes. Late changes may show recanalization of venules, centrilobular cholestasis, and an overall abnormal lobular architecture.

Risk Factors

Risk factors for VOD include

- Presence of active hepatocellular disease at the time of transplantation (increases the risk of VOD three- to fourfold)
- History of hepatitis
- Intensity of the conditioning regimen (e.g., busulfan, melphalan, radiation)
- Higher intensity of conventional chemotherapy prior to transplantation
- Acute GVHD prophylaxis (e.g., with cyclosporine *and* methotrexate)
- HLA-mismatched donor

There is no correlation, however, between any of these risk factors and the severity of VOD. The incidence of VOD seems also to be higher in patients prepared with total body irradiation, particularly those receiving a higher dose rate or total dose. VOD has been seen more often when high-dose cytosine arabinoside is added to a regimen consisting of cyclophosphamide and total body irradiation or when more than two alkylating agents (e.g., busulfan, cyclophosphamide, melphalan) are part of the conditioning regimen. Thus, VOD is more often seen in patients who are receiving a second transplant and are, for example, prepared with a combination of busulfan and cyclophosphamide (both alkylating agents). Conversely, VOD is a rare event in patients receiving a marrow transplant for aplastic anemia who have received preparation with cyclophosphamide (with or without total lymphoid irradiation) only. In some studies, the administration of cyclosporine during the preparative period together with high dose chemo/radiotherapy also seemed to be associated with an increase in the incidence of VOD. Cyclosporine and cyclophosphamide may be hepatotoxic when given individually. Cyclosporine can cause centrilobular necrosis, and cyclophosphamide has been reported to depress hepatic microsomal enzymes. Other drugs, such as dacarbazine, BCNU, 6-thioguanine and mitomycin C, have all been related to VOD. Methotrexate is generally not thought to cause hepatic problems in this setting, although it might potentiate hepatotoxic effects such as those associated with cyclosporine and alkylating agents. Older patients seem to develop VOD more often, although this has not been a consistent observation in most studies.

In patients with unexplained elevated liver function tests prior to marrow transplantation, a liver biopsy may be indicated. If this shows *active* hepatitis, it is recommended that marrow transplantation be delayed if possible until liver function tests have returned to normal, although in some cases this is not feasible due to the aggressive nature of the disease. A liver biopsy may also clarify whether elevated liver function tests are secondary to liver involvement by leukemia or lymphoma, in which case the risk of VOD is not increased and marrow transplantation should not be delayed.

Diagnosis

Signs and symptoms of VOD usually develop within 3 weeks of transplantation. Weight gain due to fluid retention and jaundice are often noticed first, followed by hepatomegaly and abdominal pain usually in the right upper quadrant. The diagnosis of VOD is likely if at least two of these features are present before day 20 post-transplant. With more severe VOD, ascites and hepatic encephalopathy may also develop. A rapidly rising bilirubin level is the worst prognostic indicator. Patients with a bilirubin 350 μmol/L (>20 mg/dL) during the first 4 weeks after the transplant have a probability of less than 10% of surviving beyond day 100. Levels of serum transaminases and alkaline phosphatase are usually only mildly or moderately elevated, and may rise later than the bilirubin. Doppler-ultrasound of the hepatic vein may show decreased or reversed flow in VOD and may be helpful to assess the extent of the disease.

Ultrasound and computed tomography may show a congested liver, ascites and the collapse of major hepatic veins. An abscess or infiltrative process can be excluded.

A liver biopsy can be useful to distinguish VOD from acute GVHD and infection of the liver as well as obstruction of hepatic veins by fungus. Since patients are generally severely thrombocytopenic early after transplantation, a percutaneous liver biopsy may be associated with an increased risk of hemorrhage. Attempts should be made to raise the platelet count to $50-60 \times 10^9$/L and maintain it at that level for ~24–36 hours after the procedure. There is also an increased risk of bleeding due to congested veins, and an associated coagulopathy. To diminish the bleeding risk, some centers prefer to perform a transfemoral or transjugular liver biopsy instead of a "blind" or ultrasound-guided procedure. The transvenous liver biopsy also permits measurement of pressure gradients between the wedged hepatic and free hepatic venous pressures. A hepatic wedge-free pressure gradient ⩾10 mmHg has a high predictive value for the diagnosis of VOD.

Differential Diagnosis

Jaundice, hepatomegaly, fluid retention and ascites may be non-specific findings (Table 22). However, their development early after transplantation (e.g., during the first week) is highly suggestive of VOD, although congestive heart failure, viral hepatitis and intra-hepatic abscess should be excluded. Jaundice together with ascites or significant weight gain (or both) are usually not seen in drug-induced hepatic cholestatic damage. Acute GVHD presents less frequently during the first 2 weeks after transplant, and usually does not present with ascites. In an occasional patient, however, symptoms of VOD may develop later and more gradually, and it might be impossible to establish an accurate diagnosis without liver histology.

Nodular regenerative hyperplasia (NRH) of the liver can present clinically with a picture very similar to VOD. It is often associated with hepatomegaly present before transplantation. Histologically, NRH will show alternating areas of atrophy and regeneration without fibrosis. Although the etiology for NRH

Table 22. Differential diagnosis of jaundice early after transplantation

	Diagnosis		
	VOD	Acute GVHD	Hepatitis
Onset (days post BMT)	0–25	>15	0–100
Bilirubin	↑ – ↑↑	↑	↑ – ↑↑
Transaminases	0– ↑	↑↑	↑↑↑
Alkaline phosphatase	↑	↑	↑↑
Weight gain	+++	–	–
Liver failure	possible	rare	possible

and VOD is probably similar, the prognosis for NRH is usually much better.

Clinical Course

VOD can present as a mild to moderately severe illness with complete recovery or as a rapidly progressive hepatic failure with encephalopathy and ensuing death. Data from the transplant center in Seattle indicate that VOD resolves in the majority of patients but contributes to death in about 30% of those who develop clinically manifest VOD. When hepatic function is significantly impaired with high bilirubin, a picture reminiscent of hepatorenal syndrome with progressive renal failure may develop. Patients with severe VOD tend to have higher peak values for bilirubin and aspartate aminotransferase as well as a more significant weight gain than patients with a mild form of VOD. Persistent jaundice along with ascites is considered a poor prognostic sign.

With an uncomplicated course, serum bilirubin and enzyme abnormalities may return to normal within 3–4 weeks. However, since acute GVHD may develop at about the same time, a delayed resolution of signs from previously diagnosed VOD can be observed. Since the therapeutic management of VOD and GVHD differ, a correct tissue diagnosis should be obtained.

Prophylaxis

Because of the possible involvement of TNF-α in the pathogenesis of VOD, the TNF-α blocker pentoxifylline is recommended starting prior to the conditioning regimen (2000 mg/day). When given prophylactically to marrow recipients, pentoxifylline lowers the TNF-α in serum, which is usually elevated in patients with VOD. Since pharmacokinetic studies have shown that high serum concentrations of busulfan are correlated with liver toxicity, dose and schedule adjustment of busulfan are generally recommended to prevent severe VOD.

Treatment

Therapeutic options are limited to symptomatic measures. A negative sodium balance should be achieved by restriction of sodium intake. All intravenous medications, including parenteral nutrition solutions, should be concentrated to reduce total volume and free water but prevent the development of a catabolic state. Concentrated dextrose solutions are preferred. Intravenous volume and renal perfusion must be maintained. Albumin (e.g., 25 g IV two to four times daily), despite its short intravascular half life, may be helpful in maintaining the serum albumin levels and the respective osmotic pressures. The hematocrit should be maintained at a level of ⩾0.30 (hemoglobin at ⩾100 g/l) with transfusion of packed red blood cells, since erythrocytes contribute to the total osmotic load and provide sufficient oxygen to hepatocytes and renal tubular cells. Spironolactone is recommended if the creatinine is <1.2 mg/dl (<100 μmol/l) and the patient can swallow the tablets. Alternatively, the use of furosemide in small doses (10–20 mg iv) in conjunction with transfusions may help maintain renal perfusion and reduce fluid retention. However, furosemide must be used cautiously, particularly in patients receiving cyclosporine (in whom renal function is already impaired). Its effect on sodium balance is also unpredictable and if used uncritically can contribute to further renal impairment. In severe VOD, hemofiltration has been used to remove volume and sodium, but generally with little success. Although the beneficial effect of low-dose dopamine (2 µg/kg/min) to increase renal blood flow is rather controversial, it is used by many centers. Low doses of heparin have likewise not been shown to have a clear beneficial effect. In addition, hemorrhagic problems are not uncommon, often necessitating dose reduction or discontinuation. Administration of tissue plasminogen activator, alone or in combination with heparin, has rapidly reversed bilirubin elevation in some patients. However, the experience at this point is limited. Prophylactic infusions of prostacyclin may be effective; unfortunately, one of the side effects of this treatment is fluid retention, with at times rather painful and edematous extremities.

Hepatic encephalopathy should be treated with oral protein restriction and possibly lactulose (side effect: diarrhea). The infusion of high-branched chain amino acid solutions is preferable to alleviate symptoms of encephalopathy, although it has no impact on the course of liver failure. Also, because of the impaired gluconeogenesis in these patients, the administration of solutions high in glucose is recommended. Protein infusions should be restricted to 50 g/day. Drugs which are predominantly metabolized by the liver, such as cyclosporine and methotrexate, need dose adjustment or must be temporarily discontinued. It is also important to use sedatives and analgesics cautiously. Due to impaired hepatic metabolism, such drugs and their metabolites can accumulate and cause an altered level of consciousness in these patients. Meperidine (Demerol®), morphine and various benzodiazepines in particular can result in a picture which may mimic hepatic encephalopathy.

Acute GVHD (see also III.2)

Pathogenesis

The cytotoxic/cytopathic effect of acute GVHD is probably the result of a combination of cellular attack (e.g., by T-lymphocytes) and the effects of cytokines such as tumor necrosis factor or interferon or others.

Histopathology

Early changes may show mild non-specific lobular hepatitis and infiltration of mononuclear cells and eosinophils in the portal triads. Intermediate changes include cholestasis, an infiltration of portal zones by lymphocytes, and destruction of small bile ducts by abnormal interlobular proliferation. Late changes can show profound cholestasis, degeneration of peripheral hepatocytes, and reduction in the number of bile ducts by abnormal interlobular proliferation.

Diagnosis

In the majority of patients, some degree of skin or intestinal involvement by acute GVHD is present concurrently, and may suggest the diagnosis of acute GVHD of the liver (see III.2). Usually the aminotransferases (transaminases) are moderately increased with only slight increase in serum bilirubin. Signs of severe liver function impairment such as acute liver failure with ascites and encephalopathy, and reduced synthesis of coagulation factors are uncommon. Especially in progressive situations, serum alkaline phosphatase may steadily increase with or without a parallel rise in bilirubin. In cases in which a differential diagnosis of VOD, hepatitis or drug-induced liver damage cannot be made with certainty, a liver biopsy needs to be performed.

Treatment

Modalities of treatment of acute GVHD are described above (III.2). With or without treatment, acute GVHD of the liver may take weeks to months to resolve completely.

Chronic GVHD (see also IV.2)

The majority of patients with chronic GVHD will show some degree of hepatic involvement, either as part of an extensive

GVHD process or as a more limited disease involving only the skin and liver. The main targets of chronic GVHD of the liver are the small interlobular bile ducts. However, the pathogenesis of their destruction and how this is immunologically mediated is largely hypothetical. Since bile duct cells express Class II histocompatibility (HLA-DR, DP, DQ) antigens, cytotoxic action of donor lymphocytes against these cells is possibly involved. Histology may show signs of active or persistent chronic hepatitis with portal inflammation and fibrosis, degeneration of bile ducts, and dense plasmacytic infiltrates in the portal area.

In the majority of cases, other organs are also affected by chronic GVHD. If the liver appears to be the only organ involved, a biopsy may be necessary to exclude other causes of hepatic dysfunction. In some patients, a persistently elevated alkaline phosphatase may represent residual damage to the intrahepatic biliary tree rather than active chronic GVHD.

Portal hypertension, hepatic failure and cirrhosis as a consequence of chronic GVHD are rare but have been observed. In two reported cases with chronic GVHD who developed hepatic failure, one had histologically proven cirrhosis and the other had an intact lobular architecture but absence of small bile ducts.

With treatment, an elevated alkaline phosphatase will usually decline within 3–4 weeks unless there is persistent damage to the biliary system. A flare-up of chronic GVHD may be heralded by increasing alkaline phosphatase levels. Prolonged treatment for 9–12 months or longer may be necessary. About half of the patients will remain free of chronic GVHD after immunosuppression is stopped. In some patients chronic GVHD of the liver may develop de novo after day 100 post marrow transplantation; in such cases the primary physician is advised to contact a transplant center to obtain information as to further management of the patient.

Both limited (confined to the liver) and extensive chronic GVHD require treatment (for details see III.2). Cyclosporine either alone or in combination with steroids has been proven to be effective. Also, thalidomide can be considered as a treatment option.

Infections of the Liver

Based on an analysis of biopsy and autopsy material, the most common infections of the liver in marrow transplant recipients are of viral etiology. Several viruses can cause hepatitis: hepatitis B or C virus, cytomegalovirus (CMV), and less often, adenovirus, varicella zoster (VZV) and herpes simplex (HSV).

Viral Infections

Hepatitis B (HBV) and C (HCV)

Although regular blood donor screening has largely eliminated HBV and to a certain extent HCV infection, it may occasionally become manifest as a reactivation of latent infection. Due to immunosuppression, patients may be unable to mount an antibody response, but may have HBV antigen or DNA in the liver. One should also keep in mind that antibodies can be positively acquired through blood transfusions and for that reason some patients may become (transiently) anti-HBs Ag or anti-HBc positive. HBs Ag carriers may be at higher risk for post-transplant fulminant hepatitis, although the reported data are not conclusive.

Using morphological criteria, hepatitis due to infection with either HBV or HCV cannot be reliably distinguished, and at times serological tests may not be accurate, since the expression of antibodies against the virus may be altered in an immunocompromised host. Liver function tests (predominantly transaminases) are variably elevated, and can fluctuate. In one series, of 17 patients who had seroconversion (from anti-HCV$^-$ to anti-HCV$^+$) after transplantation, one-half had clinical signs of active hepatitis including histological changes. It is unclear at this point how many anti-HCV$^+$ patients will develop chronic hepatitis.

Sometimes it may be difficult to distinguish between viral hepatitis and hepatic involvement by acute or chronic GVHD. If no other organs are involved, liver biopsy can be helpful in establishing the correct diagnosis and may allow institution of the appropriate therapy, although the histologic picture in chronic GVHD and chronic hepatitis may be similar, showing bile duct abnormalities along with cholestasis. Generally, a high serum alkaline phosphatase is more suggestive of chronic GVHD.

Cytomegalovirus

Infections with CMV are rather frequent, especially after allogeneic ransplantation. Usually the infection is more "generalized" and patients may have additional manifestations of a viral disease (e.g., pneumonia, marrow depression). Hepatic involvement is usually clinically less diagnostic compared to HBV or HCV infection. Histopathological alterations include multiple foci of necrosis, portal infiltrates with lymphoid cells, cholestasis and sometimes massive necrosis. Diagnosis can best be obtained through biopsy material. Although giant nuclear and cytoplasmic inclusions are typical, these are sometimes difficult to find. Monoclonal antibodies against CMV antigens together with in situ hybridization techniques may be useful in diagnosing CMV infection. However, in situ hybridization of the CMV genome cannot distinguish between active replication and persistent or latent infection. At present there is no effective treatment for these patients. The inhibitor of viral DNA replication, ganciclovir (DHPG) and the polymerase inhibitor foscarnet, either alone or in combination with high-dose CMV-hyperimmunoglobulin, are currently undergoing therapeutic trials. The use of CMV-negative blood products and prophylactic acyclovir and ganciclovir has substantially reduced the incidence of CMV disease.

Herpes Simplex Virus (HSV) and Varicella Zoster Virus (VZV)

Reactivation of herpes virus occurs in a majority of seropositive patients after transplantation, unless extended prophylaxis with acyclovir is given. The incidence can be even higher in patients with active GVHD. If the disease presents without skin involvement, liver involvement by VZV may present with abdominal pain, which can be the most prominent symptom. Liver function tests are usually elevated and patients may also have signs of pancreatitis. In severe cases, fulminant hepatic failure in the absence of or preceding a skin rash can occur. HSV and VZV viruses can be identified by immunofluorescent staining of frozen sections using monoclonal antibodies. If administered promptly, treatment with intravenous acyclovir is usually effective.

Adenovirus

Infections with adenovirus generally occur within the first 3 months after transplantation. Severe acute GVHD has been shown to be a risk factor for invasive infection, including focal hepatic necrosis, and, in an occasional patient, fulminant liver failure. Isolated liver involvement is apparently uncommon; usually the lungs, kidneys and urinary bladder (hemorrhagic cystitis or urethritis) also show signs of infection. As with HSV/VZV, diagnosis can best be obtained by immunofluorescent staining of frozen sections with monoclonal antibodies or electron microscopy.

Bacterial Infections

Bacterial infections of the liver in the form of abscesses and cholangitis are surprisingly infrequent after marrow grafting, presumably due to the early use of broad-spectrum antibiotics. However, concomitant gram-negative septicemia with moderate elevations of liver enzymes and bilirubin can occur. This may confound the diagnosis of VOD, acute GVHD, viral infection, or drug induced liver damage which may be present concurrently.

Fungal Infections

Hepatic involvement by fungi occurs in at least half of the patients with disseminated fungal infection. Most commonly, *Candida albicans* and *tropicalis* are involved but other species such as *Candida parapsilosis*, *stellatoidea* or *krusei* are occasionally found. Usually fungal cultures from extrahepatic sites (stool, urine, oropharynx) are positive. *Aspergillus* species cause a more fulminant clinical picture, preferentially involving different organs (lungs, brain, paranasal sinus); liver involvement is often documented only at autopsy. Other fungi such as *Trichosporum cutaneum* or *Histoplasma capsulatum* are found less frequently.

Fungal infections of the liver may present as cysts, granulomas, multiple small abscesses and obstruction of biliary ducts by fungus balls. Obstruction of hepatic veins may mimic VOD. Patients often will have persistent fever, liver tenderness and an elevation of alkaline phosphatase. Ultrasound, computed tomography and guided find needle aspiration should be performed to obtain the diagnosis.

Drug-Induced Hepatic Damage

Cyclosporine

Cyclosporine is extensively metabolized in the liver and subject to biliary elimination. The serum half-life increases as serum bilirubin increases: in one study in patients with no, mild, and moderate hepatic dysfunction the corresponding half-life values were 3.5, 5.8 and 8.7 hours. It is therefore recommended that the cyclosporine dose be reduced if the bilirubin increases.

Cyclosporine can induce a centrilobular hemorrhagic necrosis, and the simultaneous administration of cyclosporine along with preparative chemo/radiotherapy can increase liver toxicity. This has also been reported in patients with aplastic anemia who developed severe VOD when cyclosporine was given during the pre-transplant preparative period. Observations in renal transplant patients, in whom no GVHD occurs, indicate that cyclosporine frequently causes a moderate rise in bilirubin and, less often, transaminases. Alkaline phosphatase may be only slightly elevated.

The incidence of transient liver function abnormalities is higher when cyclosporine is combined with methotrexate. Cyclosporine toxicity can often be distinguished from hepatic GVHD by its onset early post-transplant, the rate of rise of serum bilirubin (usually mild), and confirmation of high cyclosporine blood levels, although this relationship is not always observed. If liver toxicity develops later, it may be impossible to identify the underlying cause without additional diagnostic procedures.

Methotrexate

Although elevations of transaminases are commonly seen after higher doses of intravenous methotrexate, no significant histopathologic changes in the liver have been described with the low-dose prophylactic regimen (10–15 mg/m^2 IV or IT) used in the setting of marrow transplantation. However, in combination with other hepatotoxic drugs that may be part of the conditioning regimen or post-transplant cyclosporine, methotrexate may add toxicity and should be withheld if the bilirubin increases significantly.

Azathioprine

This drug is occasionally used to treat active chronic GVHD. Since it can cause an increase in alkaline phosphatase and transaminases, a liver biopsy may be helpful to distinguish liver toxicity from chronic GVHD. Findings such as bile duct lesions or "ductopenia" are more consistent with chronic GVHD.

Parenteral Nutrition

Long-term parenteral nutrition can cause cholestatic hepatitis and hepatomegaly due to fatty changes and water accumulation. Jaundice is usually mild and liver function tests may be slightly elevated. Due to a lack of regular gallbladder contractions, dilatation of the bladder and bile stasis can occur in these patients. This can predispose to acalculous cholecystitis, and occasionally obstruction of the cystic duct, manifested in the form of biliary colic. If long-term parenteral nutrition is required, it is usual to give lipids intermittently (e.g., 3 times per week) or alternate parenteral and oral feeding.

Recurrent Malignancy

Although a rare event, this possibility should be considered particularly in patients transplanted for the treatment of malignant lymphoma. Usually ultrasound, computed tomography and liver biopsy are helpful in obtaining the diagnosis quickly.

References

Ayash LJ, Hunt M, Antman K, Nadler L, Wheeler C, Takvorian T, Elias A, Antin JH, Greenough T, Eder JP (1990) Hepatic venoocclusive disease in autologous bone marrow transplantation of solid tumors and lymphomas. J Clin Oncol 8:1699

Beschorner WE, Pino J, Boitnott JK, Tutschka RJ, Santos GW (1980) Pathology of the liver with bone marrow transplantation. Effect of busulfan, carmustine, acute graft versus host disease and cytomegalovirus infection. Am J Pathol 99:396

Dulley FL, Kanfer EJ, Appelbaum FR, Amos D, Hill RS, Buckner CD, Shulman HH, McDonald GB, Thomas ED (1987) Venoocclusive disease of the liver after chemoradiotherapy and autologous bone marrow transplantation. Transplantation 43:870

Jones RJ, Lee KSK, Beschorner WE, Vogel VG, Grochow LB, Braine HG, Vogelsang GB, Sensenbrenner LL, Santos GW, Saral R (1987) Venoocclusive disease of the liver following bone marrow transplantation. Transplantation 44:778

Locasciulli A, Bacigalupo A, Vanlint MT, Tagger A, Uderzo C, Portmann B, Shulman HM, Alberti A (1991) Hepatitis C virus infection in patients undergoing allogeneic bone marrow transplantation. Transplantation 52:315

Locasciulli A, Bacigalupo A, Van Lint MT, Chemello L, Pontisso P, Occhini D, Uderzo C, Shulman HM, Portmann B, Marmont AM, Alberti A (1990) Hepatitis B virus (HBV) infection and liver disease after allogeneic bone marrow transplantation: A report of 30 cases. Bone Marrow Transplant 6:25

McDonald GB, Sharma P, Matthews DE, Shulman HM, Thomas ED (1985) The clinical course of 53 patients with venocclusive disease of the liver after marrow transplantation. Transplantation 39:603

McDonald GB, Sharma P, Matthews DE, Shulman HM, Thomas ED (1984) Venocclusive disease of the liver after bone marrow transplantation: Diagnosis, incidence, and predisposing factors. Hepatology 4:116

McDonald GB, Shulman HM, Sullivan KM, Spencer GD (1986) Intestinal and hepatic complications of human bone marrow transplantation. Part I. Gastroenterology 90:460

McDonald GB, Shulman HM, Sullivan KM, Spencer GD (1986) Intestinal and hepatic complications of human bone marrow transplantation. Part II. Gastroenterology 90:770

Menard DB, Gisselbrecht C, Marty M, Reyes F, Chumaeaux D (1980) Antineoplastic agents and the liver. Gastroenterology 78:142

Roslyn JJ, Pitt HA, Mann LL, et al. (1983) Gall bladder disease in patients on long-term parenteral nutrition. Gastroenterology 84:148

Shulman HM, Hinterberger W (in press) A review of the hepatic venocclusive disease – liver toxicity syndrome after bone marrow transplantation. Bone Marrow Transplant

Snover DC, Weisdorf S, Bloomer J, McGlave P, Weisdorf D (1989) Nodular regenerative hyperplasia of the liver following bone marrow transplantation. Hepatology 9:443

Yee GC, Kennedy MS, Storb R, Thomas ED (1984) Effect of hepatic dysfunction on oral cyclosporine pharmacokinetics in marrow transplant patients. Blood 64:1277

7. Kidneys and Urinary Tract

Overview

In contrast to the liver, the kidneys are less frequently the primary target of a pathological event after bone marrow transplantation. Acute and chronic GVHD do not obviously affect the kidney, although some cases of nephrotic syndrome possibly related to GVHD have been reported. A specific disease entity related to chemo/radiotherapy-induced damage has not been observed; however, it is likely that a subclinical degree of tubular damage occurs during the conditioning regimen. Renal impairment is predominantly secondary to circulatory disturbances associated with VOD, septicemia or hypovolemic shock, or is related to drugs frequently used post-transplant that can injure the tubular system (such as cyclosporine and amphotericin). In general, the severity of renal impairment can range from mild pre-renal insufficiency to acute oliguric (or anuric) renal failure. Furthermore, hemorrhagic cystitis secondary to drug toxicity or infections can occur in up to 30% of all transplant recipients and can cause significant morbidity and mortality after marrow transplantation.

Renal Insufficiency Secondary to Circulatory Problems

This syndrome is often a consequence of intravascular volume depletion and associated hypotension. Common causes are capillary leak syndrome, severe gastrointestinal losses and septic shock. In severe cases, pre-renal insufficiency may lead to acute oliguric renal failure. Treatment should be directed at maintaining sufficient intravascular volume by infusion of albumin and red cells, correction of electrolyte imbalances and dose reduction of potentially nephrotoxic drugs such as cyclosporine, amphotericin B and aminoglycoside antibiotics (see below).

Pre-renal insufficiency due to circulatory imbalance must be distinguished from a catabolic state, which usually shows a disproportional rise of serum urea compared to relatively normal serum creatinine. Proteins and dietary calories should be given freely if renal function abnormalities are due to a severe catabolic state, but should be restricted in pre-renal insufficiency.

In severe cases of pre-renal insufficiency or toxic damage, acute renal failure secondary to acute tubular necrosis can develop—particularly when nephrotoxic drugs are given at the same time. Most of these patients will have a high output failure with subsequent oliguria. Common causes include nephrotoxins such as cyclosporine, aminoglycosides, amphotericin B, prolonged hypotension or the hepatorenal syndrome in the course of severe VOD. Some patients may require temporary hemodialysis. Because of the high protein requirements of patients after transplantation, amino acids should be administered routinely. Non-protein calories can be supplied by concentrated dextrose (i.e., 25% or greater) and lipids. Furthermore, it is advisable to keep the hemoglobin at a high level ($>100 \text{ g/l}$) to provide sufficient oxygen to the kidney and to increase the intravascular oncotic pressure. Although somewhat controversial, some centers also give "low doses" of continuous dopamine infusion ($2 \mu\text{g/kg/min}$) to improve renal blood flow. The prognosis with renal function impairment secondary to pre-renal insufficiency is usually rather good; after the underlying disease has been corrected with appropriate drug dose adjustment and supportive measures, kidney function can recover completely.

Drug-Induced Renal Toxicity

Although several antineoplastic drugs such as CCNU, mitomycin and adriamycin are nephrotoxic, no significant nephrotoxicity has been associated with the drugs commonly used in the preparative regimen before marrow grafting. However, these drugs might cause sub-threshold damage to the kidney which can lead to exaggerated responses with other agents. Most of the potentially nephrotoxic drugs such as cyclosporine, various antibiotics, antifungal and antiviral agents are employed in the post-transplant period.

Aminoglycosides

Aminoglycosides are frequently given after bone marrow transplantation as treatment or prophylaxis of infections with gram negative bacteria. However, they are nephrotoxic in a dose-related fashion as they accumulate in the liposomes of proximal tubular cells, where they are bound to phospholipids. This may lead to (usually reversible) focal necrosis and interstitial proliferation. The degree of nephrotoxicity seems to vary between different aminoglycosides and it appears that amikacin is the least nephrotoxic compound.

Cyclosporine

Nephrotoxicity of cyclosporine is associated with renal vascular injury, most likely due to inhibition of prostacyclin synthesis in the epithelial vascular cells. Histologically, vascular injury with arteriolar and glomerular capillary thrombosis as well as interstitial sclerosis can be seen. Early signs of kidney damage from cyclosporine can consist of proteinuria, bicarbonate loss, impaired urinary concentrating ability and urinary casts.

Some renal function impairment during cyclosporine treatment can be expected in a high proportion of patients, who will develop an elevated serum creatinine level $\geqslant 50\%$ above baseline within days of starting cyclosporine. Volume depletion, additional nephrotoxic drugs, hepatic dysfunction (especially VOD), septicemia and prolonged hypotension are associated with a more rapid rise in creatinine. In particular, aminoglycosides and amphotericin B given concurrently with cyclosporine can increase nephrotoxicity significantly. The same is true for trimethoprim-sulfamethoxazole, as it interferes with tubular secretion of creatinine. In marrow transplant patients, renal dysfunction is usually reversible after withdrawal of cyclosporine, even in patients who have had elevated serum creatinine levels for several months. However, if severe renal damage has occurred, recovery might not be complete and chronic renal damage may persist. Chronic renal failure has been described repeatedly in cardiac transplant recipients on long-term cyclosporine.

If renal dysfunction develops in patients on cyclosporine therapy, some drug adjustments are recommended:

1. When creatinine rises markedly (50% over previous day's value), 1–2 doses of cyclosporine should be withheld, hydration should be increased and other nephrotoxins should be dose-adjusted or discontinued, if possible.
2. When creatinine rises gradually, the dosage should be reduced by at least 25%. In general, it is advisable to try to give the drug at a reduced level rather than withhold it.
3. If the creatinine is between 1.5 mg/dl and 2.0 mg/dl (132–177 µmol/l), the daily dose should be reduced by approximately 50% and doses given adjusted to the serum level.
4. If the creatinine exceeds 2.0 mg/dl (177 µmol/l), cyclosporine should be held.

The role of serum or blood cyclosporine levels in monitoring drug-related renal toxicity is controversial. Even high levels over a long period of time may not necessarily be associated with significant renal impairment. Many investigators agree that the most practical approach is careful monitoring of serum creatinine and blood urea nitrogen levels as indicators of renal damage requiring adjustment of cyclosporine dose to maintain a serum level of 200–300 mg/ml.

Acyclovir

Renal damage can occur when acyclovir is given at higher doses, especially if the patient is not sufficiently hydrated. Crystal formation in the renal tubules, the collecting ducts, or both have been described. When the drug is administered by slow infusion over 1 h along with adequate hydration, the incidence of raised blood urea nitrogen and creatinine levels should be lower. However, if renal failure develops in a transplant patient and creatinine clearance is below 50 ml/min, a dose reduction is required. The same is true for ganciclovir (DHGP) used for prophylaxis and treatment of CMV infections.

Cyclophosphamide

Hemorrhagic cystitis is a serious side-effect of high-dose cyclophosphamide therapy in marrow transplant patients. It is caused by a urotoxic metabolite of cyclophosphamide, acrolein, and typically begins during the first few days after infusion. It can persist for several months. Its incidence can be reduced by forced diuresis (200–250 ml/h in adults) with or without bladder irrigation. Some centers give mesna (2-mercaptoethane sulfonate sodium) concomitant with the cyclophosphamide infusion; it is administered intravenously (160% of the cyclophosphamide dose) and is rapidly excreted via the urinary tract. Within the urinary tract, mesna combines with acrolein to form a non-toxic compound. The timing of mesna administration seems to be important (before and then 3, 6 and 9 hours after cyclophosphamide, or alternatively as a continuous infusion), and timing errors may result in a loss of its protective effect. It is of note, however, that mesna was not shown to be superior to hydration in a recent randomized study. It may have its indication in patients in whom the fluid balance is a concern. Despite these preventative measures, about 30% of patients receiving cyclophosphamide will nonetheless develop cystitis.

In addition to cyclophosphamide, etoposide and busulfan at higher doses can occasionally cause hemorrhagic cystitis; this can be prevented by forced diuresis for at least 3 days after the drugs have been stopped.

Treatment options for hemorrhagic cystitis are limited. At times it can be quite painful for the patient, requiring spasmolytic or analgesic drugs or both. The use of intravesical prostaglandin E_2 has been reported to be of benefit in some patients; however, to be effective it must be retained in the bladder for some time, which can likewise be painful for some patients. Continuous bladder hydration should be given via a Foley catheter, especially when clots are formed and urethral obstruction is a concern. Some urologists recommend that alum be added to the hydration fluid. Some patients may absorb hydration fluid through the damaged bladder mucosa and can present with symptoms of fluid overload (pulmonary edema) or even alum "intoxication". Some patients with severe persistent cystitis may require cauterization of bleeding mucosa with formaldehyde via cystoscopy.

It should be pointed out that the course of hemorrhagic cystitis can vary greatly. Some patients experience a short period of hematuria following chemotherapy administration. In others, it occurs with some time-lag and may manifest itself, for example, when the patient develops severe thrombocytopenia. Hemorrhagic cystitis occuring later after transplantation is thought to be due to viral infection.

Delayed problems after resolution of the acute cystitis are rare. However, an occasional patient may develop bladder spasms or be plagued by reduced bladder capacity.

Infections

In general, infectious complications of the kidney are not very frequent after marrow transplantation; in particular, bacterial infections such as pyelonephritis are very rarely encountered. Kidney involvement often occurs as part of a systemic infection, and renal impairment can develop as a consequence of bacteremia and septic shock. However, about 5–10% of autopsied marrow recipients show involvement of the kidney with fungus. The most common organisms found are *Candida sp*. Abscess formation has been described.

CMV can cause severe and often fatal infections of the lung and liver; however, for unknown reasons, CMV does not primarily affect the kidney, although urinary excretion is not infrequent.

If hemorrhagic cystitis develops on a delayed basis after marrow transplantation, other (specifically, viral) causes must be considered. Probably due to the more profound immunodeficiency and propensity toward viral infections, hemorrhagic cystitis due to viral infection is more often seen after allogeneic than after autologous BMT. Virus cultures sometimes fail to give a positive result and it has been suggested that thin-sectioning of urinary sediment (showing viral inclusion bodies) should be utilized. Affected patients sometimes have some neutrophil or platelet count depression, suggesting a more systemic viral infection.

In a series of about 1000 transplanted patients, adenovirus could be isolated from the urine of 10%. Most patients with hemorrhagic cystitis or kidney infection due to adenovirus also have signs of disseminated disease involving organs such as lung, gut and liver. Polyomavirus has also been identified in the urine of affected patients. It is not clear whether infection with polyomavirus can also cause infections of other organs such as the lung or liver.

Treatment options for adeno- and polyomavirus infections are limited. If the patient is receiving post-transplant immunosuppression, and acute GVHD is not active, a dose reduction of immunosuppressive drugs might be considered. Vidarabine is being used experimentally. In addition, polyvalent immunoglobulins can be given intravenously, since these preparations generally contain antiviral titers. It should be noted, however, that no data are available as to the efficacy of these measures.

Microangiopathic Hemolytic Anemia (MAHA)

This clinical syndrome is characterized by the occurrence of hemolytic anemia due to red blood cell fragmentation, renal insufficiency and consumptive thrombocytopenia. Its etiology is still unclear; factors such as radiation-induced damage to the kidney ("radiation nephritis") and cyclosporine have been implicated. The latter is believed to cause inhibition of synthesis of prostacyclins in endothelial cells which are potent inhibitors of (local) coagulation. Active GVHD is often present, and the syndrome is more frequent after unrelated-donor transplants. The laboratory diagnosis is made if schistocytes are seen on the blood film. Frequently, the serum LDH and bilirubin are increased and the haptoglobin is decreased.

Depending on the degree of hemolysis, patients may require frequent blood and platelet transfusions. The syndrome is usually quite resistant to treatment; decreasing the dose of cyclosporine or stopping the drug completely can help to control the extent of hemolysis, and plasmapheresis is occasionally of benefit, but heparin has been shown to be ineffective.

References

Ambinder RF, Burns W, Forman M, Charache P, Arthur R, Beschorner W, Santos G, Saral R (1986) Hemorrhagic cystitis associated with adenovirus infection in bone marrow transplantation. Arch Intern Med 146:1400

Arthur RR, Shah KV, Baust SJ, Santos GW, Saral R (1986) Association of BK viruria with hemorrhagic cystitis in recipients of bone marrow transplants. N Engl J Med 315:230

Atkinson K, Biggs JC, Golovsky D, Concannon A, Dodds A, Downs K, Ashby M (1991) Bladder irrigation does not prevent haemorrhagic cystitis in bone marrow transplant recipients. Bone Marrow Transplant 7:351

Hiraoka A, Ishikawa J, Kitayama H, Yamagami T, Teshima H, Nakamura H, Shibata H, Masaoka T, Ishigami S, Taguchi F (1991) Hemorrhagic cystitis after bone marrow transplantation: Importance of a thin sectioning technique on urinary sediments for diagnosis. Bone Marrow Transplant 7:107

Holler E, Kolb HJ, Hiller E, Mraz W, Lehmacher W, Gleixner B, Seeber C, Jehn U, Gerhartz HH, Brehm G, Wilmanns W (1989) Microangiopathy in patients with cyclosporine prophylaxis who developed acute graft-versus-host disease after HLA-identical bone marrow transplantation. Blood 73:2018

Kennedy MS, Deeg HJ, Siegel M, Crowley JJ, Storb R, Thomas ED (1983) Acute renal toxicity with combined use of amphotericin B and cyclosporine after marrow transplantation. Transplantation 35:211

Shepherd JD, Pringle LE, Barnett MJ, Klingemann H-G, Reece DE, Phillips GL (1991) Mesna versus hyperhydration for the prevention of cyclophosphamide-induced hemorrhagic cystitis in bone marrow transplantation. J Clin Oncol 9:2016

Shields AF, Hackman RC, Fife KH, Corey L, Meyers JD (1985) Adenovirus infections in patients undergoing bone-marrow transplantation. N Engl J Med 312:529

Shulman H, Striker G, Deeg HJ, Kennedy M, Storb R, Thomas ED (1981) Nephrotoxicity of cyclosporin A after allogeneic marrow transplantation. N Engl J Med 305:1392

Shurafa M, Shumaker E, Cronin S (1987) Prostaglandin F_2-alpha bladder irrigation for control of intractable cyclophosphamide-induced hemorrhagic cystitis. J Urol 137:1230

Van Why SK, Friedman AL, Wei LJ, Hong R (1991) Renal insufficiency after bone marrow transplantation in children. Bone Marrow Transplant 7:383

8. Central Nervous System

Overview

The spectrum of CNS complications after marrow transplantation is notable for lack of direct involvement of the brain (in contrast to many other organs) by acute GVHD. The following major CNS complications have been observed:

- Leukoencephalopathy
- Drug-induced neurotoxicity
- Infections
- Hemorrhage
- Recurrence of malignancy
- Metabolic encephalopathy

Since the symptomatology of these entities is very similar, a computerized tomography (CT-) scan of the brain as well as a lumbar puncture should be performed to help establish the diagnosis. Specimens of the cerebrospinal fluid should be examined for number and type of cells and the presence of microorganisms (gram stains for bacteria, silver and india ink stains for fungus, and Ziehl Neelson for *Mycobacterium tuberculosis*), and for protein and sugar; bacteriologic cultures, virus isolation and cryptococcal antigen tests should be performed.

Before a lumbar puncture can be safely performed, a low platelet count must be corrected; usually at least 30×10^9/L platelets are recommended. Furthermore, a lumbar puncture carries some risk if the pressure of the cerebrospinal fluid is high, for it increases the possibility of a fatal cerebellar or tentorial pressure cone.

Leukoencephalopathy

Pathogenesis

The combined application of CNS irradiation at doses of ≥ 20 Gy and intrathecal chemotherapy can result in irreversible brain damage. These modalities act synergistically in the sense that radiation apparently alters the blood-brain barrier and allows the intrathecal drug improved access to the central nervous system.

Intrathecal methotrexate has most often been described as being associated with the development of this complication. The role of intrathecal cytarabine in the development of leukoencephalopathy is not clear, probably because it has been given together with radiation less often than has methotrexate. However, considering the potential neurotoxic effects of this drug, the frequency of leukoencephalopathic changes can be anticipated to be similar to that seen with the use of methotrexate.

Histopathology

Demyelinization is accompanied by multifocal to confluent non-inflammatory necrosis; dystrophic calcification and ventricular dilatation can also be seen.

Risk factors for the development of leukoencephalopathy include pre-transplant CNS therapy or prophylaxis with irradiation, intrathecal chemotherapy or both, a preparative regimen containing total body irradiation, and the administration of several courses of intrathecal methotrexate post-transplant.

Post-transplant leukoencephalopathy is most frequently seen in patients with acute lymphoblastic leukemia who have received cranial or craniospinal irradiation and intrathecal chemotherapy, or both, as CNS prophylaxis during their induction/consolidation therapy. The risk of developing leukoencephalopathy is around 5–10% in such patients, and might be higher in the pediatric age group. A conditioning regimen containing total body irradiation along with post-transplant methotrexate on its own does not appear to increase the risk of this complication in children who have not previously been given CNS prophylaxis or therapy.

The manifestations of leukoencephalopathy are not strictly age-related. The fact that it is apparently seen more often in young patients might be more related to the age distribution of acute lymphoblastic leukemia.

The overall risk of developing leukoencephalopathy is lower than the risk of CNS relapse when post-transplant intrathecal methotrexate is omitted. In one study among patients with a history of CNS disease, the probability of CNS relapse was 52% in patients who did not receive intrathecal methotrexate compared to 17% in those who received this post-transplant prophylaxis. For patients who had no CNS disease before marrow grafting, the corresponding figures were 19% and 4%, respectively. There is some evidence that a lower dose of post-transplant methotrexate administered via an Omaya reservoir may lower the risk of neurotoxicity.

Diagnosis

Symptoms can be non-specific and may include lethargy, slurred speech, ataxia, seizures, confusion, dysphagia, spasticity, dementia and decerebrate posturing. As an early sign, CT-scans of the brain may show a decreased density, which may be reversible; later, destruction of the white matter, ventricular dilatation and calcification may be seen. Myelin basic protein and enolase levels are elevated in the CNS fluid during the acute phase and may be used to monitor patients or help in the differential diagnosis. Nuclear magnetic resonance imaging (MRI) may establish a diagnosis of cerebral lesions earlier and more reliably than is possible with a conventional CT-scan.

Clinical Course

Symptoms of leukoencephalopathy usually become manifest during the first month after transplantation and may sometimes progress to a severe, irreversible clinical picture. From experience with conventional treatment of leukemia, it is known that early leukoencephalopathy-associated changes may be reversible when chemo/radiotherapy affecting the brain is stopped in time. However, no such information is available for transplanted patients.

A delayed form of neurotoxicity may become obvious later (i.e., months to years) after marrow grafting. This is most often seen in patients who received combined radiation/intrathecal methotrexate before the age of 3 years. Histopathology shows white matter necrosis and dystrophic calcification of the small vessels. Symptoms are forgetfulness, confusion and poor performance at school (specifically, difficulties with reading and arithmetic).

Differential Diagnosis

Meningeal leukemic involvement can create a blockage of cerebrospinal fluid drainage and may cause symptoms and signs of increased intracranial pressure. CT-scan and lumbar puncture usually establish the diagnosis, and also help to differentiate leukoencephalopathy from infectious and bleeding complications of the brain.

Treatment

Leukoencephalopathy is a degenerative process, and no effective therapy is available; therefore, pre-transplant therapy should be planned with a view toward preventing this complication. One can, for instance, consider alternative conditioning regimens not including total body irradiation for patients at risk; determination of myelin basic protein in cerebrospinal fluid can possibly identify such high-risk patients. In any case, no more than five doses of intrathecal methotrexate should be given after transplantation, since data suggest that there is no added benefit from more than this number irrespective of CNS leukemia status at transplantation.

Drug-Induced Neurotoxicity

The spectrum of neurotoxic drugs used before and after marrow transplantation is limited.

Cytosine Arabinoside (Ara C)

High-dose Ara C (1.5–3 g/m^2 for several days) is part of various preparative regimens. Neuropathy is a serious complication with this drug, and must be distinguished from leukoencephalopathy, infection, bleeding and leukemia of the CNS. Histologically one can see damage or loss of Purkinje cells from the lateral hemisphere along with proliferation of astrocytes. Since about 40–60% of the Ara C plasma concentration can be found in the cerebrospinal fluid, and CNS toxicity is related to the dose administered and not to the duration of exposure, the incidence of CNS symptoms increases significantly at a cumulative dose of over 36 g/m^2. However, occasional symptoms may develop at lower doses if the patient has been treated with high-dose Ara C before transplantation (e.g., during remission induction therapy). Symptoms usually develop within 6–8 days after the first dose and may include personality changes, disturbances in the level of consciousness, headache, somnolence, confusion, scomatoma, paraplegia, cerebellar toxicity, and occasionally seizures. Symptoms are reversible within a few days after stopping the drug. However, cerebellar ataxia and dysarthria may be irreversible in about 10% of all such patients.

Busulfan

This drug is part of the frequently-used "BuCy" conditioning regimen. Busulfan can enter the cerebrospinal fluid, achieving concentrations similar to those in plasma, and can be found for some 24 hours after discontinuation. Generalized seizures have been described and prophylaxis with phenytoin is recommended; a loading dose (18 mg/kg/day) one day prior to starting busulfan should be given and the drug continued according to serum levels (usually a dose of 100 mg three times daily is sufficient) until at least 48 hours after the last dose of busulfan. It is important to achieve a therapeutic phenytoin level as seizures can occur with suboptimal levels. Diazepam is occasionally given instead as it achieves a faster steady-stage concentration and has fewer pharmacological interactions.

Cyclosporine

Patients receiving this drug can present with a variety of neurological symptoms. Cyclosporine neurotoxicity has been associated with urinary retention, ataxia, drowsiness, mental confusion and quadriparesis. Some of the neurological symptoms (in particular grand mal and focal seizures, tremor, depression and cerebellar ataxia) have been linked to a low level of serum magnesium which is caused by renal wasting secondary to cyclosporine-induced tubular damage. Regular magnesium replacement may prevent some of these neurological complications. However, not all neurological side effects are clearly linked to a low magnesium level; there seems to be a direct effect of cyclosporine on the CNS, facilitated by accumulation of cyclosporine and its metabolites in the cerebrospinal fluid secondary to a defective blood-brain barrier. There is also no clear link to an elevated plasma or serum cyclosporine level. In some cases, the concurrent administration of cyclosporine and high-dose methylprednisolone has been suspected to be causative. Children seem to be more susceptible to the toxic neurological effects of cyclosporine (particularly, seizures). It has also been suggested that cyclosporine neurotoxicity is more often seen in patients transplanted for a hematologic malignancy, but rarely in patients who have received a transplant for aplastic anemia. It may be possible that the neurotoxicity is cumulative, with cyclosporine, intrathecal methotrexate and total body irradiation all contributing.

Cortical blindness is often heralded by visual disturbances and can progress within a few hours to complete blindness. Occipital lobe density changes may be seen on CT-scan or MRI. Risk factors for this complication are ill-defined but there seems to be a predisposition in those patients who have developed microangiopathic hemolytic anemia (MAHA). It is possible that cyclosporine induces endothelial damage (characterized by microangiopathic blood changes) and can also cause vascular cerebral damage leading to local platelet aggregation. Cortical blindness is usually reversible after discontinuation of cyclosporine. Some authors recommend prophylactic phenytoin in those patients who have signs of underlying MAHA.

A coarse tremor is rather common in patients receiving cyclosporine and is not predictive of any further neurological side-effects. In some patients, grand mal tremor of the upper extremities can occur. In an occasional patient, mental depression will be the only sign of cyclosporine neurotoxicity and will disappear when the drug is stopped. Hand and foot pain occurring during cyclosporine infusion has occasionally been reported; this symptom is most likely caused by the diluent used for the intravenous cyclosporine preparation, although a contribution by GVHD is possible.

Descriptions of the pathological changes associated with cyclosporine neurotoxicity are rare. However, cyclosporine plays a role in the pathogenesis of vascular lesions by inhibiting vascular prostacyclin synthesis. This may lead to microthrombi and focal necrosis. There are some case reports implicating a disturbance of the blood-brain barrier due to cyclosporine, leading to bile staining edema and focal necrosis of the brain.

Acyclovir

Approximately 1% of patients receiving intravenous acyclovir develop encephalopathic changes characterized by lethargy, obtundation, tremors, confusion, hallucinations, agitation, seizures or coma; this has been reported with both parenteral and oral administration, and particularly in patients with renal failure. Acyclovir should also be used with caution in patients who have shown neurological side-effects from other neurotoxic drugs (e.g., Ara C, cyclosporine) or those receiving concomitant intrathecal methotrexate. The potential neurotoxic effects of acyclovir seem to be dose-related and a level between 0.14 to 1.2 μg/ml is considered safe. Moreover, if a patient develops renal failure, serum levels can increase and cause neurological symptoms.

Ganciclovir

Neurological side-effects similar to those observed with acyclovir have been reported for ganciclovir, including irritability, confusion, loss of hearing and seizures.

Steroids

Steroids are part of most prophylactic and therapeutic protocols for acute and chronic GVHD. Side-effects are dependent on the dose and the duration of the treatment. Neurological complications can manifest as headache, psychosis, vertigo, convulsions and increased intracranial pressure (pseudotumor cerebri).

Infections

Generally, because of the less profound and complex immunodeficiency after autologous bone marrow transplantation, infections of the CNS occur less often in that setting than after allogeneic transplantation.

Fungi

The most frequent infections of the CNS are due to fungi. Although *Aspergillus* and *Candida* are the most common pathogens, a number of infections with "rare" fungi such as mucor have been reported more recently.

Aspergillus

CNS involvement in the form of brain abscess is relatively common in patients who have disseminated aspergillosis. *Aspergillus* species are primarily respiratory pathogens, and consequently the majority of infections involve either the sinus or the lungs. In about 30% of patients, however, the infection disseminates throughout the body since *Aspergillus* has a propensity for invading blood vessels. The rhino-cerebral form originates in the sinuses and progresses through soft tissues, cartilage, and bone, causing lesions in the palate and the nose. Occasionally, the infection progresses through the base of the skull to involve the brain. Amphotericin B is the only antifungal agent with established activity against *Aspergillus sp.*; it has been combined with 5-fluorocytosine and rifampin, but there is no conclusive evidence that these combinations have any advantages over Amphotericin B alone. Experience with newer antifungal drugs (e.g., itroconazole) is limited.

Candida

Hematogenous dissemination of *Candida* (*C. albicans*, *tropicalis*, *krusei*) may manifest with retinal abscesses, symptoms of which include orbital pain, blurred vision, scotoma and opacities. Meningitis and brain abscesses occur in about 20% of patients with disseminated infection. The diagnosis may be difficult to establish because only non-specific abnormalities may be found in the cerebrospinal fluid, and the fungus may not be seen or successfully cultured.

Cryptococcosis

This fungus is less common after marrow transplantation than *Aspergillus* and *Candida*. *Cryptococcus* is ubiquitous in animals and soil specimens; in humans, infections begin in the lungs, where in normal persons it may remain asymptomatic and resolve without therapy. Dissemination can occur in patients after marrow transplantation, and a regular feature is central nervous system infection which may manifest as meningoencephalitis. Early symptoms include headache, nausea, staggering gait, irritability, confusion, and blurred vision. Fever and nuchal rigidity are usually mild or absent. A chest x-ray may disclose a dense infiltrate if pulmonary cryptococcosis is also present; primary lesions are present in about 10% of affected patients. A lumbar puncture is the most useful test, and an India ink smear may reveal encapsulated yeast. A test for crytococcal antigen may be positive. The most definitive test, however, is the culture.

Bacteria

Post-transplant meningitis due to bacteria is a rare event and may occur later after marrow grafting, predominantly in patients who have developed chronic GVHD and require continuous immunosuppressive treatment. *Pneumococcus*, *meningococcus*, *Hemophilus influenzae* and *Klebsiella pneumoniae* are the most common pathogens. The manifestations are those of any acute pyogenic meningitis and include chills, fever, headache, nuchal rigidity, delirium and cranial nerve palsies. Brain abscesses from *Staphylococcus aureus* are occasionally seen. If bacterial infection of the CNS is suspected, the spinal fluid should be investigated. With appropriate chemotherapy, recovery can be expected in two-thirds of all cases.

Viruses

Viral infections of the CNS are infrequent after marrow grafting. Many patients are placed on prophylactic acyclovir after transplantation and therefore CNS infections with herpes virus are uncommon. However, specifically in patients who are not receiving proper prophylaxis with acyclovir, or in those with chronic GVHD, *herpes simplex* (HSV) or disseminated *varicella zoster* infection can be the cause of encephalitis which may present with a range of neurological symptoms. HSV type I can ascend from the respiratory epithelium of the nose up the olfactory tract to reach the frontal and temporal areas of the brain. In the cerebrospinal fluid, a lymphocytosis and elevated protein content may be found as fairly nonspecific alterations. Early diagnosis can best be obtained by MRI in combination with an electroencephalogram; a CT-scan of the brain will usually not show signs of focal necrosis before the third day of infection. The only definitive means of diagnosing HSV encephalitis is the isolation of HSV by brain biopsy. Treatment with intravenous acyclovir or ganciclovir can be effective when started in time (i.e., before the onset of coma), and full recovery may occur.

Toxoplasmosis

Although rare, reactivation of quiescent infection (cysts) with liberation of toxoplasmosis trophozoites may occur virtually anywhere throughout the body. However, about 50% of transplanted patients with fatal toxoplasmosis have signs and symptoms of encephalitis and more than 90% also have pathological evidence of brain involvement. Neurological signs can be highly variable and may include disturbances of consciousness, motor impairment, diffuse meningoencephalitis, cerebellar ataxia and seizures.

Serologic tests may be insensitive in patients lacking immune response. However, *toxoplasma gondii* can be isolated from the peripheral buffy coat cells and inoculated on human fibroblast cultures. A cytopathic effect is seen in an infected individual after 2–3 weeks. In addition, the CNS fluid can have some characteristic features such as mononuclear pleocytosis and pronounced elevation in protein along with normal glucose. For treatment, pyrimethamin should be given with a loading dose of 2 mg/kg for the first 2 days; in severe infections, doses can be doubled and given every day. In addition, sulfadiazine is recommended at a dose of 100 mg/kg/day.

Hemorrhage

Hemorrhagic complications of the CNS are not very frequent since patients are usually given prophylactic platelet support to maintain a level of about $20 \times 10^9/L$. Even in allosensitized recipients, a low platelet count is frequently tolerated without hemorrhage, as due to the usual age limit for marrow transplantation most patients would not be expected to have an underlying degenerative process of the vascular system. However, the situation is different if the patient is septic and has concomitant coagulation abnormalities or suffers from high blood pressure. In an occasional patient, hemorrhage may also be seen as a complication of CNS fungal infection, most often *aspergillus*. In any event, CT-scan or MRI of the brain along with a lumbar puncture will allow the diagnosis to be obtained quickly.

Recurrence of Malignancy

CNS recurrence of malignancy is relatively infrequent in patients given a marrow transplant for acute myelogenous

Table 23. Intrathecal Methotrexate After Marrow Transplantation

Diagnosis:
  Acute myelogenous leukemia in remission or relapse
  Chronic myelogenous leukemia in chronic phase or blast crisis of myeloid type
  Non-Hodgkin's lymphoma, low-grade histology

Recommendations:
  Diagnostic lumbar puncture pre-transplant and injection of one dose of methotrexate
  If cerebrospinal fluid is negative for leukemic cells, no further methotrexate to be given
  If there is evidence of leukemia, one additional dose of methotrexate pre-transplant and four doses post-transplant to be given

Diagnosis:
  Acute lymphoblastic leukemia in remission or relapse
  Chronic myelogenous leukemia in blast crisis of lymphoid type
  Non-Hodgkin's lymphoma, aggressive histology

Recommendations:
  Diagnostic lumbar puncture pre-transplant and injection of one dose of methotrexate
  If cerebrospinal fluid is negative for leukemic cells, no further intrathecal methotrexate pre-transplant; if positive, one additional dose of methotrexate to be given pre-transplant
  All patients to be given four doses of intrathecal methotrexate post-transplant

leukemia or chronic myelogenous leukemia in chronic phase. However, it does occur in a fraction of patients transplanted for acute lymphoblastic leukemia or some high-grade lymphomas; in these patients, CNS relapse often heralds bone marrow relapse. Therefore, post-transplant methotrexate is recommended for these patients regardless of previous chemo/radiotherapy of the brain and spine. Apparently there is no added benefit from more than five doses of post-transplant methotrexate or Ara C irrespective of CNS leukemia status at transplant. Table 23 summarizes the current recommendations for CNS prophylaxis with methotrexate after marrow grafting for various malignancies.

Neurological symptoms of CNS malignancy are usually nonspecific. Analysis of cerebrospinal fluid, CT-scan and MRI imaging can help to distinguish CNS relapse from infectious or bleeding complications.

Metabolic Encephalopathy

Renal or hepatic failure of various etiologies can cause encephalopathy. Symptoms may vary from mild disturbances of the level of consciousness to coma. If there is no obvious correlation of these symptoms to renal/hepatic dysfunction, other transplant-related complications must be excluded by CT-scan and lumbar puncture.

References

Barrett AJ, Kendra JR, Lucas CF, et al. (1985) Disturbance of blood-brain barrier after bone marrow transplantation. Lancet 2:280

Cohen SMZ, Minkove JA, Zebley III JW, Mulholland JH (1984) Severe but reversible neurotoxicity from acyclovir. Ann Intern Med 100:920

Eck P, Silver SM, Clark EC (1991) Acute renal failure and coma after a high dose of oral acyclovir. N Engl J Med 325:1178

Ghany AM, Tutschka PJ, McGhee Jr RB, Avalos BR, Cunningham I, Kapoor N, Copelan EA (1991) Cyclosporine-associated seizures in bone marrow transplant recipients given busulfan and cyclophosphamide preparative therapy. Transplantation 52:310

Grigg AP, Shepherd JD, Phillips GL (1989) Busulphan and phenytoin. Ann Intern Med 111:1049 [Correction in: Ann Intern Med 112:313 (1990)]

Lazarus HM, Herzig RH, Herzig GP, Phillips GL, Roessmann U, Fishman DJ (1981) Central nervous system toxicity of high-dose systemic cytosine arabinoside. Cancer 48:2577

Reece DE, Frei-Lahr DA, Shepherd JD, Dorovini-Zis K, Gascoyne RD, Graeb DA, Spinelli JJ, Barnett MJ, Klingemann H-G, Herzig GP, Phillips GL (1991) Neurologic complications in allogeneic bone marrow transplant patients receiving cyclosporin. Bone Marrow Transplant 8:393

Rubin AM, Kang H (1987) Cerebral blindness and encephalopathy with cyclosporin A toxicity. Neurology 37:1072

Shepp DH, Hackman RC, Conley FK, Anderson JB, Meyers JD (1985) *Toxoplasma gondii* reactivation identified by detection of parasitemia in tissue culture. Ann Intern Med 103:218

Thompson CB, June CH, Sullivan KM, Thomas ED (1984) Association between cyclosporin neurotoxicity and hypomagnesaemia. Lancet 2:1116

Thompson CB, Sanders JE, Flournoy N, Buckner CD, Thomas ED (1986) The risks of central nervous system relapse and leukoencephalopathy in patients receiving marrow transplants for acute leukemia. Blood 67:195

Tollemar J, Ringden O, Ericzon B-G, Tyden G (1988) Cyclosporine-associated central nervous system toxicity. N Engl J Med 318:788

IV. Delayed Transplant Related Problems

1. Follow-Up after Discharge from the Transplant Center

Patients who are discharged from a transplant center to return to the care of their primary physician usually look back on a period of at least 3–4 months of intensive medical and psychological care. Being "discharged" for many patients is frightening and they respond by regression.

Every transplant team has developed its own approach to these problems. At the pretransplant evaluation, the patient must have a clear understanding that transplantation is aimed at cure and never palliation. Consequently, once the procedure has been completed the goal must be rehabilitation. The aim of any bone marrow transplant, be it allogeneic, syngeneic or autologous, is to return the patient to a productive life. To allow for a smooth transition from the protected environment of a transplant unit to daily routine on the outside will require a sensitive approach by physicians, nurses, social workers and other support staff. This transition will begin at the transplant center and will continue under the care of the patient's referring physician.

While being cared for at a transplant unit, the patient will have been seen by physicians or nurses at least once or twice weekly after discharge and occasionally every day. A thorough evaluation (Table 24) is carried out before the patient is discharged from the transplant center, about three months after transplantation. After discharge home the patient should be seen at least once weekly for the first month. If no new medical problems develop and the patient is stable these intervals can be lengthened to two weeks for the next two months and eventually to three weeks or monthly intervals, depending on the patient's clinical status. It appears useful to obtain a chest x-ray at the time the patient is first seen at home, and to monitor liver function tests, complete blood counts as well as food intake and weight regularly.

Table 24. Studies for longterm evaluation

– Physical examination	– Gynecological evaluation
– Complete blood count	– Endocrinologic evaluation
– Chemistry survey	Growth hormone
– Creatinine clearance	Thyroid function
– Chest radiograph	Sex hormones
– Ophthalmologic evaluation	– Pulmonary function tests
– Oral medicine evaluation	– Disease restaging
– Marrow aspiration	
Cytology	
Chimerism studies	

Table 25. Delayed Complications

– Marrow dysfunction	– Infertility
– Immunodeficiency	– Cataracts
– Chronic GVHD	– Aseptic necrosis
– Infection	– Dental problems
– Autoimmune disorders	– Genitourinary dysfunction
– Pulmonary disease	– Secondary malignancy
– Neuroendocrine dysfunction	– Intellectual impairment
– Impaired growth	– Psychological problems

As an increasing number of patients have been followed now for up to two decades, it has become apparent that numerous delayed complications can develop (Table 25). Several reviews have recently been published. Some major problem areas are discussed below and in subsequent chapters.

Immune Function and Daily Activities

High doses of chemotherapy and total body irradiation given at the time of marrow transplantation are intended not only to eradicate the patient's underlying disease but also to suppress the patient's immune system such that the donor marrow can successfully engraft. Consequently, all transplant recipients are subject to a prolonged period of immunodeficiency which is most severe during the first three to five months. At the time the patient is discharged from the transplant center, the period of highest risk of bacterial, fungal and viral infections has been overcome. However, it will take at least 5-6 months, even in patients who do not have any serious complications e.g., chronic GVHD, for immune functions to gradually improve and return to normal. In patients with chronic GVHD abnormalities persist for much longer.

Thus, a major concern after the patient's discharge is that of infection. Some transplant teams, therefore, recommend that the patient continue to wear a surgical mask for at least six months. This is aimed at reducing the risk of infections due to certain microorganisms, viruses and fungi. It is likely, however, that the screening effect of these masks is minimal. Nevertheless, they appear to be useful as a reminder to patients that their immune function has not yet returned to normal, and that they are constantly at risk of infection. It is important for patients to avoid contact with individuals suffering from viral infections such as measles, German measles, chicken pox, and varicella zoster. Conversely, hand washing is more important than wearing the face mask.

Most viral infections occur during the first 2-3 months after transplant (III.4), but some present later. Varicella zoster has been observed in approximately half of all bone marrow transplant recipients within the first year of grafting. As agents such as acyclovir have become available, most patients are being treated with a 7 to 10 day course of parenteral acyclovir. The responses to acyclovir are generally excellent; however, 10-15% of patients may have disease recurrence, presumably due to the fact that the development of anti-viral immunity is prevented by early anti-viral therapy. For patients who are inadvertently exposed to shingles or chicken pox within the first year of transplantation and have not had a recent infection, zoster immune globulin (ZIG) should be given, starting within six days of exposure. Usually ZIG can be obtained via the Red Cross or other regional blood centers.

Interstitial pneumonia, like other viral infections, usually occurs within the first 2-3 months after transplantation (III.5). If a patient develops a clinical picture of respiratory distress, with hypoxemia and radiographic findings of diffuse pulmonary interstitial infiltrates after returning home, the center where the patient was transplanted should be contacted so that appropriate management can be discussed.

The attitude towards a return to normal activities will vary from patient to patient even in the absence of any significant medical problems. In general, patients should be encouraged to gradually expand their activities, and to keep physically and mentally active. Nevertheless, caution is indicated and a patient should not return to work or to school for at least 6 or possibly 9 months following transplantation. Most patients will easily comply with this since they often seem to lack the energy necessary to carry a full work load. It will also take some time for the patient to regain a normal appetite and enjoy food, which will allow him to consume the amount of calories necessary for normal performance. Food intake often increases with the return of salivary secretion, and a recovery of smell and taste sensation.

There should be little concern about household pets, plants, or garden work; patients should stay away from compost heaps and similar places which contain a high concentration of aspergillus spores. Caution is recommended in any contact with barnyard animals (because of fungal diseases and parasites), and swimming in public or private pools should be avoided because of the high frequency of heavy contamination with potentially pathogenic organisms. In any event, whenever outside for work or leisure, patients should use sun blocking creams to prevent actinic triggering or reactivation of chronic GVHD (see below). Patients may resume normal sexual activity but constraint in the number of sexual partners is recommended. Of course, recommendations in regard to "safe sex" apply to transplant patients as they do for healthy individuals. Vaginal dysfunction may be present, however, due to hormone deficiency or chronic GVHD.

Hematologic Function

Engraftment of donor cells usually occurs within 2–3 weeks of transplantation and granulocyte counts of $1 \times 10^9/1$ or greater are reached within one month of transplantation. Consequently, the patient no longer requires antibiotic coverage (III.4) other than trimethoprim/sulfamethoxazole which is given 2 days/ week for long term prophylaxis. Similarly, most patients are independent of platelet transfusions within 4–6 weeks of transplantation. It is rare that platelet transfusions are required beyond day 100, i.e., at the time the patient usually returns to the care of the referring physician. In patients given ABO incompatible transplants a reticulocytopenic anemia may persist for some time. If transfusions are required they should be irradiated, at least during the first 6 months after transplantation, with approximately 2000 cGy in vitro to prevent the occurrence of transfusion-induced GVHD. Recently, several cases of hemolytic uremic syndrome have been observed many months after transplant, at times associated with cyclosporine tapering (see III.7).

Another potential problem is marrow graft rejection. In contrast to transplantation of solid organs such as kidney or liver, where acute or chronic rejection are frequent problems, rejection is a relatively infrequent event in marrow transplantation. Although some cases of rejection with or without autologous recovery have been observed late after transplantation, most occur early. This problem is discussed in detail elsewhere (III.3).

Any change in hematological parameters should be investigated, not only from the point of view of graft failure, but also in regard to the possibility of recurrence of an underlying malignancy. A fall in leukocytes or platelets in peripheral blood might also be due to other reasons including viral infections, progression of chronic GVHD, or myelosuppression by treatment for chronic GVHD with azathioprine. In any event, if changes occur, a work-up including bone marrow aspiration and possibly biopsy should be obtained. If recurrent leukemia is suspected, it is helpful to also have available marrow slides obtained at the time the patient's original diagnosis was established. Furthermore, if a marrow aspirate is obtained, samples should be secured for cytogenetic analysis, particularly in patients in whom the donor was of different sex or when the original leukemia had an identifiable chromosomal marker. If there was no sex difference, a sample to be analyzed for restriction fragment length polymorphism or by other molecular biology techniques to determine donor or host origin should be obtained. In more than 95% of cases the recurrence of leukemia will be of the original host type. In the remaining cases, however, either a new leukemia in host-derived cells or a leukemia occurring in donor cells, either of the same phenotype or a phenotype different from the original leukemia may be observed. Most recurrences of leukemia following marrow transplantation will occur within 1–2 years of transplantation, but recurrences as late as 6 or 8 years following transplantation have been observed. In any case of recurrence, it is advisable to notify the center at which the patient was transplanted.

Since in some respects marrow transplantation is still an experimental procedure, the request by most transplant centers that the patient return for a thorough reevaluation, approximately one year and possibly even later after transplantation, seems appropriate. Since new problems are constantly being recognized and, more importantly, new methods of treatment are being established, optimum treatment can probably be provided only by an experienced team.

References

Deeg HJ (1990) Early and late complications of bone marrow transplantation. Current Opinion In Oncology 2:297–307

Hows J, Palmer S, Gordon-Smith EC (1985) Cyclosporine and graft failure following bone marrow transplantation for severe aplastic anemia. Br J Haematol 60:611–617

Loughran TP, Jr., Sullivan K, Morton T, Beckham C, Schubert M, Witherspoon R, Sale G, Sanders J, Fisher L, Shulman H, Thomas ED, Storb R (1990) Value of day 100 screening studies for predicting the development of chronic graft-versus-host disease after allogeneic bone marrow transplantation. Blood 76:228–234

Lum LG (1990) Immune recovery after bone marrow transplantation. Hematol/Oncol Clin North Am 4:659–675

Nims JW (1991) Survivorship and rehabilitation. In: Whedon MB (ed), Bone Marrow Transplantation, Principles, Practice and Nursing Insights. Boston: Jones & Bartlett, Boston 334–345

Smith CI, Aarli JA, Biberfeld P, Bolme P, Christensson B, Gahrton G, Hammarstrom L, Lefvert AK, Lonnqvist B, Matell G, Pirskanen R, Ringden O, Svanborg E (1983) Myasthenia gravis after bone-marrow transplantation – Evidence for a donor origin. N Engl J Med 309:1565

Sniecinski IJ, Oien L, Petz LD, Blume KG (1988) Immunohematologic consequences of major ABO-mismatched bone marrow transplantation. Transplant 45:530–534

Sullivan KM (1991) Special care of the allogeneic marrow transplant patient. In: Wiernik PH, Canellos GP, Kyle RA, Schiffer CA (eds), Neoplastic Diseases of the Blood, 2nd ed. Churchill Livingstone, New York 933–947

Wingard JR, Curbow B, Baker F, Piantadosi S (1991) Health, functional status, and employment of adult survivors of bone marrow transplantation. Ann Intern Med 144:113–118

2. Chronic Graft-Versus-Host Disease

Etiology

Chronic GVHD typically develops >3 months post-transplant, although histologic and clinical manifestations can be present earlier. Chronic GVHD differs from acute GVHD in its distribution of target organs and clinical presentation. T-lymphocytes are likely involved in the pathogenesis of both types, but in contrast to acute GVHD, in which T-cells respond to alloantigens, T-cells in chronic GVHD react in an autoimmune fashion against histocompatibility alloantigens of the host (public determinant of MHC class II molecules). These T-cells produce abnormal patterns of cytokines and can stimulate the production of collagen by fibroblasts. In long-term stable survivors without chronic GVHD, alloimmunity seems to be blocked by specific suppressor cells which usually are not found in patients with chronic GVHD. It has also been postulated that the establishment of tolerance requires a functioning thymus. Since thymus function can be impaired as a consequence of chemo/radiotherapy or acute GVHD, the lack of thymus function may hamper the development of specific suppressor cells capable of mediating stable graft-host tolerance, and/or delete autoreactive T-cells. The donor-host directed alloaggression may be only an initial event leading to autoimmune symptoms, impaired immune reconstitution and infections and it is likely that the release of certain cytokines contributes to the manifestation of chronic GVHD.

Clinical Manifestations

Most patients developing chronic GVHD will have had preceding acute GVHD. Symptoms develop usually within 2 years of transplantation, either as a *progressive* extension of acute GVHD or following a quiescent period after resolution of acute GVHD. In addition, about 20–30% of patients will have *de novo* late-onset GVHD without evidence of prior acute GVHD. Studies have shown that the prognosis is poorest in those patients who have the progressive-onset type (Fig. 7).

With the exception of the skin, it is unusual to have chronic GVHD isolated to a single site. The spectrum of clinical symptoms resembles several known collagen vascular diseases such as scleroderma, systemic lupus erythematosus, lichen planus, Sjogren's syndrome, rheumatoid arthritis and primary biliary cirrhosis (Fig. 8). In contrast to several of these disorders, however, renal and CNS involvement is not seen in chronic GVHD. A clinicopathological classification according to the extent of organ involvement has been developed which allows the discrimination between *"limited"* and *"extensive"* chronic GVHD (Table 26). *"Subclinical"* chronic GVHD is defined as the presence of characteristic pathology on both skin and oral biopsies without clinical signs or symptoms of chronic GVHD.

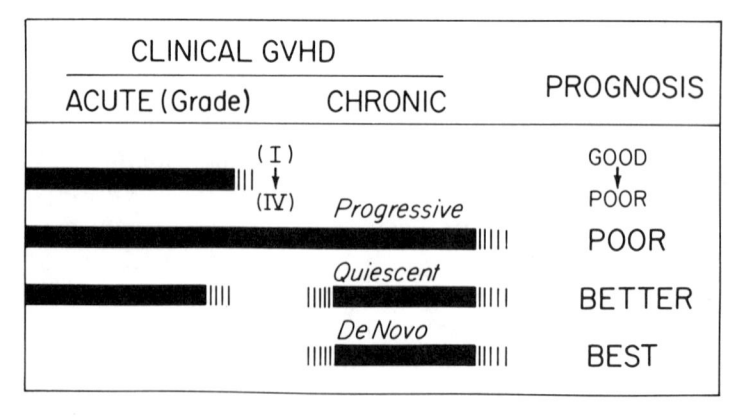

Fig. 7. Presentation of chronic GVHD relative to acute GVHD, as progressive, quiescent or *de novo* form

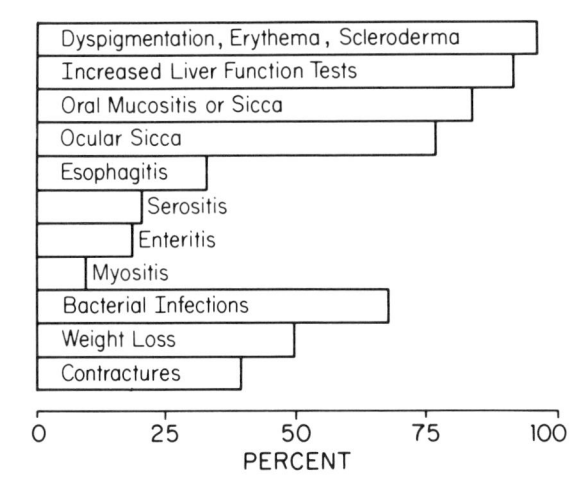

Fig. 8. Incidence of clinical manifestations in patients with extensive chronic GVHD. (Reprinted with permission from H.J. Deeg et al., Bone Marrow Transplantation: A Review of Delayed Complications. Br. J. Haematol (1984) 57:185)

Table 26. Clinicopathological classification of chronic graft-versus-host disease

---

Subclinical graft-versus-host disease:
  Histologically positive but no clinical symptoms
Limited chronic graft-versus-host disease:
  Either or both:
  – Localized skin involvement
  – Hepatic dysfunction (due to chronic GVHD)
Extensive chronic graft-versus-host disease:
  Either:
  – Generalized skin involvement;
  or
  – Localized skin involvement or hepatic dysfunction due to chronic GVHD or both, plus:
  – Liver histology showing chronic aggressive hepatitis, bridging necrosis, or cirrhosis; or
  – Involvement of eye (Schirmer's test with less than 5 mm wetting); or
  – Involvement of minor salivary glands or oral mucosa demonstrated on labial biopsy; or
  – Involvement of any other target organ (lung, kidney)

Adopted and modified from Shulman and colleagues.

Skin

The skin is involved in more than 95% of patients who develop chronic GVHD. Early symptoms include dryness, itching and absence of sweating, while later on tightness and contracture may develop. Raynaud's phenomenon is not common. Nail abnormalities, patchy alopecia, dyspigmentation and mucous membrane abnormalities, in particular dryness, are frequent (Table 27).

Table 27. Skin manifestations of chronic GVHD

Early:	– Erythema with macules and plaques
	– Desquamation
	– Dyspigmentation
	– Vitiligo
	– Leukoderma
	– Lichen planus-like lesions
	– Nail abnormalities
	– Alopecia
Late:	– Induration
	– Contractures
	– Atrophy
	– Poikiloderma

The onset of skin symptoms is usually gradual. However, in some cases, chronic GVHD of the skin can evolve with an intense inflammatory phase with edematous areas and desquamation after minimal trauma or sun (UV-light) exposure. Lichen planus-like lesions can sometimes herald a flare of skin GVHD. Inadequately-treated patients develop progressively indurated skin which is fixed to the underlying fascia. Clinically the picture resembles scleroderma, with atrophic epidermis, thickened dermis and poikiloderma. A brown-coloured patchy hyperpigmentation, joint contractures and skin ulcerations may complete the picture (Fig. 9).

Histopathologically, two major types of skin GVHD can be distinguished. The first is the *generalized* type, which is characterized by epidermal hypertrophy and hyperkeratosis, clusters of eosinophilic bodies, and an increasing thickening of the basement membrane and the papillary dermis.

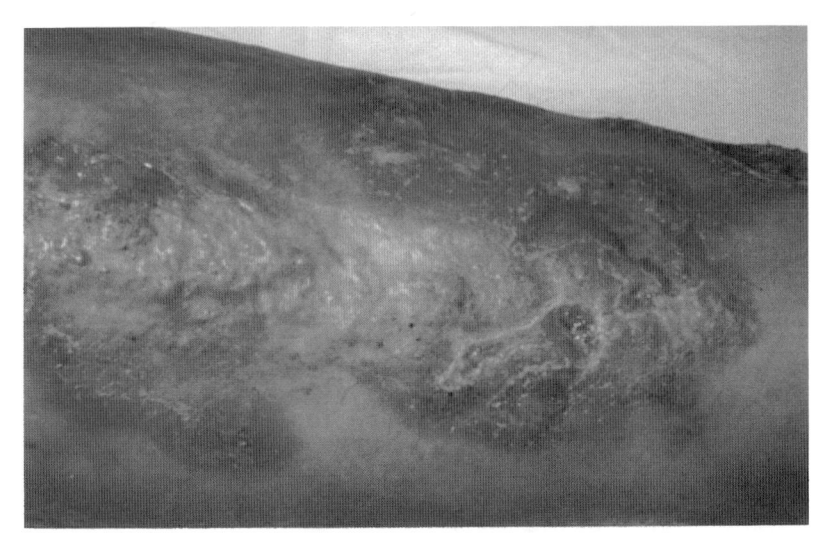

Fig. 9. Chronic GVHD of the skin after protracted course, with atrophy of the epidermis, induration of the dermis and ulcerations (sclerodermalike changes)

Immunoglobulin (IgM) and complement deposits can be found at the dermal-epidermal junctions of cutaneous lesions. With localized chronic GVHD, lichenoid reactions with eosinophilic bodies are rarely seen. Instead, dense focal dermal fibrosis and epidermal atrophy occur without any significant inflammation.

Mouth

Like skin involvement, involvement of the mouth is seen in a large proportion (>70%) of patients with extensive chronic GVHD. The most frequent symptoms are pain (particularly with spicy and hot foods) and dryness of the mucous membranes (sicca syndrome). Lichen planus-like lesions of the buccal and labial mucosa are common (Fig. 10) and can easily be misdiagnosed as oral candidiasis. Xerostomia may lead to dental caries, periodontitis and atrophy of the filiform papillae. In more severe forms, ulcerations can occur. Histopathological changes include atrophy, necrosis of squamous cells and

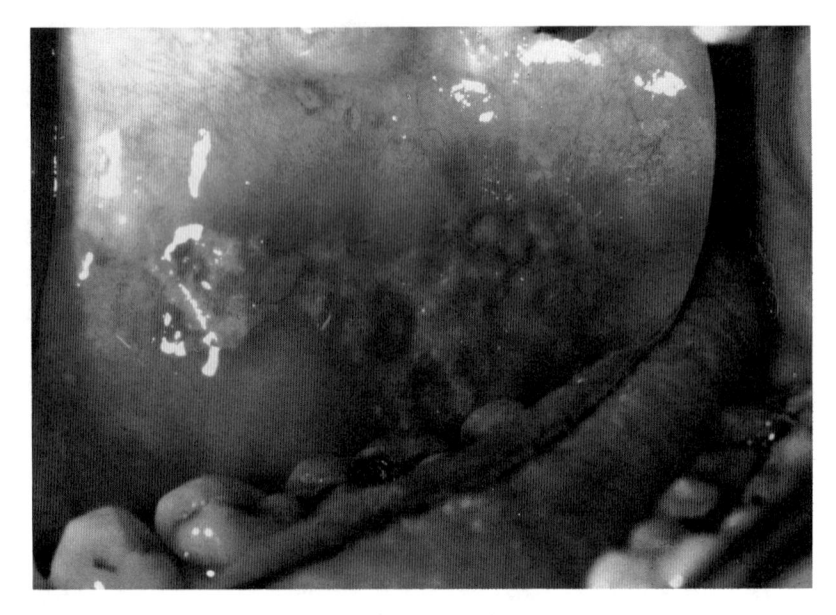

Fig. 10. Chronic GVHD of the oral mucosa, showing typical lichen planus-like changes. There is also neovascularization best, visible in the upper part of the picture

mononuclear cell infiltration characteristic of a lichenoid reaction. Salivary glands may show a lymphoplasmacytic cell infiltration around the ducts, ultimately leading to fibrosis of the gland.

Eyes

Ocular involvement is observed in up to 80% of patients with extensive chronic GVHD. Most of the symptoms develop secondary to insufficient tear production as part of the sicca syndrome of chronic GVHD, which may cause pain, burning, blurring and photophobia. Ocular sicca can also lead to keratitis and scarring. Histologic review reveals tarsal and conjunctival inflammation along with lacrimal gland fibrosis. Although less frequent, the uvea can also be involved by chronic GVHD: iritis, iridocyclitis and choroiditis can occur, and reflect the "autoimmune" character of chronic GVHD. To assess the extent of lacrimal insufficiency, a Schirmer's test is recommended. Pathological changes of the cornea (keratitis sicca) need evaluation by fluorescein biomicroscopy. Patients with "dry eyes" should use artificial tears to prevent progressive corneal erosion, perforation or scarring. When assessing eye involvement by chronic GVHD, it should be remembered that total body irradiation and long-term use of corticosteroids can cause ocular problems, in particular cataract formation (see IV.5). In addition to the mouth and eyes, sicca syndrome can also involve the genital tract, particularly the vagina, and the mucosa of the tracheobronchial tree.

Gastrointestinal Tract

Intestinal involvement is less common with chronic than with acute GVHD. Pathologic changes are most often seen in the esophagus, where it can present as dysphagia, pain, swelling or retrosternal pain. "Web formation" associated with mucosal desquamation, strictures and partial occlusion, along with functional abnormalities can be diagnosed by barium esophagogram, and are localized mainly in the upper esophagus (Fig. 11). This must be considered a late syndrome occurring mainly in insufficiently treated patients. Endoscopy may reveal epithelial peeling or desquamation. Manometric studies have shown a spectrum of motility disorders ranging from aperistalsis to high amplitude contraction. In contrast to scleroderma, esophageal muscle fibrosis is not characteristic of chronic GVHD. Problems arise when the esophageal involvement causes symptoms such as dysphagia which may lead to poor caloric intake and weight loss. Esophageal obstruction can also cause aspiration and subsequent recurrent pulmonary disease. In order to prevent irreversible changes, it is important to recognize chronic GVHD of the esophagus early in its course and initiate appropriate immunosuppressive treatment.

About 90% of all patients with chronic GVHD also have various degrees of chronic liver disease. The outcome is usually more favorable when it is associated with skin manifestations only ("limited" chronic GVHD) than in patients with extensive

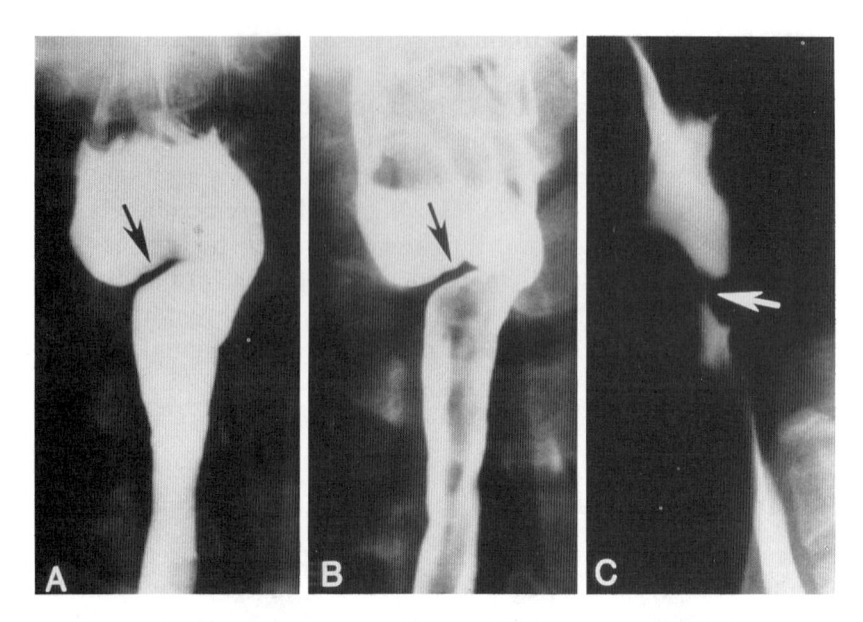

Fig. 11. Chronic GVHD of the esophagus. Radiograph of a barium swallow in an inadequately treated patient showing web formation and partial occlusion. (Reproduced with permission from G.B. McDonald et al., "Radiographic features of esophageal involvement in chronic graft-vs-host disease", Am. J. Roentgenol (1984) 142:501

chronic GVHD. Pathology and clinical picture of this complication are described in more detail in III.6.

In contrast to acute GVHD, the stomach and intestinal tract are rarely affected by chronic GVHD. In a screening program conducted in Seattle, only a few patients showed signs of chronic GVHD of the gut. Patients may at times have some diarrhea, crampy abdominal pain or both. Malabsorption can occur, mainly related to fibrotic changes in the lamina propria, submucosa and mucosa.

Vagina

Extensive chronic GVHD may involve inflammation, sicca, adhesion and stenosis of the vagina. If chronic GVHD is not active, factors such as sequelae of total body irradiation, inappropriate hormone replacement and atrophy due to inactivity should be considered. If atrophy is the most likely cause, dilators and estrogen creams are recommended. If chronic GVHD is suspected to be significantly contributing to vaginal problems, systemic immunosuppressive treatment is necessary. In some cases surgical intervention may be required.

Serosal Involvement

Some degree of serosal involvement is encountered in about 10–20% of patients with extensive chronic GVHD that is insufficiently treated. Symptoms are secondary to pericardial, pleural and synovial effusions.

Lung

Obstructive lung disease has been increasingly recognized as a late manifestation of chronic GVHD. About 10–20% of long-term survivors with chronic GVHD may ultimately develop this type of complication, which is presumed to be "triggered" by viral infections and can be quite resistant to treatment. Its clinical features are described in more detail in IV.3.

Diffuse pulmonary fibrosis has also been seen occasionally in patients with chronic GVHD. Histologically, some of these patients have lymphocytic bronchitis and lymphocytic infiltrations of the lung interstitium. Chest x-ray shows interstitial pneumonitis, and open lung biopsy is recommended to obtain the characteristic histology and to rule out infections.

Neuromuscular Complications

Several patients with chronic GVHD have been described as meeting the diagnostic criteria for myasthenia gravis, including the distribution of muscular weakness, response to edrophonium, repetitive nerve stimulation and antibodies against the acetylcholine receptor; symptoms appeared late after transplant as corticosteroid therapy was being tapered. It is not clear which patients with chronic GVHD are at risk of developing myasthenia gravis. Other rare neuromuscular abnormalities in chronic GVHD may include polymyositis and peripheral neuropathy.

Autoimmune Problems

The clinical manifestations of chronic GVHD resemble those of some spontaneous autoimmune diseases. However, the autoantibody profile is significantly different. Antinuclear antibodies can be found in up to 80% of patients after marrow transplantation, without any difference between patients with and without chronic GVHD. Antibodies against nuclear antigen (native DNA and nuclear antigen) are usually negative. Antibodies against mitochondria, epidermal cells and smooth muscle cells are also occasionally found. However, the presence of any of these autoantibodies can not be correlated with clinical symptoms, except in some patients with GVHD who develop anti-platelet antibodies that can cause autoimmune thrombocytopenia. This idiopathic thrombocytopenic purpura (ITP)-like syndrome may require specific treatment including steroids and splenectomy in resistant cases.

Immunodeficiency

Patients with chronic GVHD have delayed immune recovery and usually remain immunodeficient as long as the disease is active. Both B- and T-lymphocytes can be quantitatively and qualitatively altered. Specifically, the percentage of suppressor cells remains increased along with a decreased number of helper cells. Helper cells usually produce a variety of cytokines, which support function and interaction of specific immune cells. In B-cells, the response to neo-antigens is delayed along with the ability of B-cells to switch from IgM production to IgG production in secondary responses. A long lasting IgG subclass deficiency has also been reported (predominantly IgG_2 and IgG_4), predisposing the patient to infections with gram-positive bacteria.

In addition, patients with chronic GVHD often have a deficiency of intestinal secretory immunity and a reduced level of salivary IgA, particularly if sialadenitis is also present. This secretory IgA deficiency may contribute to the frequent sinobronchial infections observed in patients with chronic GVHD. In addition to disorders of the specific immune response, functions involving the nonspecific immune system such as granulocyte chemotaxis and opsonin activity of monocytes are also defective.

The pathogenesis of the delayed recovery of immune function in patients with chronic GVHD has not yet been sufficiently delineated. Some studies suggest that the normal maturation of T-cells is interrupted by specific blockages at one or more levels after grafting. Since the thymus plays a central role in educating lymphoid cells and is usually destroyed by acute GVHD and the preparative regimen, this lack of thymic education might contribute to the immunodeficiency in patients with chronic GVHD.

Diagnosis and Grading

The diagnosis of chronic GVHD is based on clinical and histopathological criteria, and pathological assessment is needed. A punch biopsy should be obtained from the involved skin. Even in the absence of a skin rash, a biopsy from the sun-exposed forearm can show diagnostic changes. Histopathological criteria for active skin disease include basal vascular degeneration, eosinophilic body formation, and lymphoplasmacytic cell infiltration.

In addition, an oral biopsy from the inner lower lip (approximately 5 mm long and 3 mm deep) should be obtained to establish and stage the activity of chronic GVHD. If biopsies are positive for GVHD without any clinical symptoms, the chronic GVHD is "subclinical". Other sites that may require histological confirmation are the liver, esophagus, lung and muscle. Table 28 summarizes diagnostic procedures recommended to establish the diagnosis of "limited" or "extensive" clinical chronic GVHD. The severity of chronic GVHD and its impact on the patient is best graded by Karnofsky performance status (Table 29).

Predictive Factors

Factors which have been shown to be associated with an increased incidence of chronic GVHD include:

Table 28. Diagnostic procedures to assess activity and organ involvement of chronic GVHD

Screening Study	Abnormality
In all patients:	
Skin biopsy from forearm	Eosinophilic bodies, basal vacuoles
Oral/lip biopsy	Mucositis, sialadenitis, IgA bearing plasma cells
Schirmer's test	≤5 mm wetting
Slit lamp examination	Corneal stippling
Liver function tests	Elevated
Pulmonary function tests	Forced midexpiratory flow decreased, FEV/FVC decreased
Recommended if symptoms are present:	
Upper GI endoscopy with biopsy	"Web" formation, strictures
Barium swallow (x-ray)	Desquamative esophagitis
Lower GI endoscopy with biopsy	Degeneration of glands, fibrosis of lamina propria, submucosa and serosa
Malabsorption tests	Stool fat increased

Table 29. Karnofsky score

(%)	Description
100	Normal, no complaints; no evidence of disease.
90	Able to carry on normal activity; minor signs or symptoms of disease.
80	Normal activity with effort; some signs or symptoms of disease.
70	Cares for self and is well but unable to work. Requires infrequent outpatient follow-up and sees M.D. only once a week.
60	Requires occasional assistance but is able to care for most needs. Visits M.D. 2–3 times a week.
50	Requires considerable assistance and frequent medical care. Daily or alternate-day M.D. visits are necessary.
40	Disabled and requires special care. If outpatient, requires special M.D./R.N. care; if inpatient, requires little active care (up, out of bed and in good condition).
30	Severely disabled and hospitalization is indicated although death is not imminent. Clinical condition is fair.
25	Hospitalization is mandated. Condition is fair to poor, but stable.
20	Active supporting treatment in hospital is required. Condition is poor and unstable.
15	Active intensive care is continually required. Condition is critical.
10	Patient is moribund with a fatal process rapidly progressing. Condition is thought to be hypercritical.
5	Patient is moribund. Condition is terminal and irreversible. ("No code" status.)
0	Patient is dead.

- Preceding acute GVHD
- Greater patient age
- Non-HLA-identical transplant
- Infusion of non-irradiated donor buffy-coat cells after transplantation for aplastic anemia
- Second marrow infusion for poor graft function

In a recent study, 19% of long-term survivors with previous acute GVHD Grades 0-I developed chronic GVHD, compared to 57% of survivors with Grades II-IV acute GVHD. About 70% of recipients of unrelated-donor marrow will develop chronic GVHD, usually earlier after transplantation than occurs with matched sibling-donor transplant. Most centers assess the activity of chronic GVHD based on studies around 3 months post-transplant ("day 100 workup") (Table 28), and decide whether or not prolonged immunosuppressive treatment is required. In particular a positive skin or oral biopsy has a high predictive value: of those patients in whom this is the only sign of chronic GVHD (subclinical chronic GVHD), about 70% will develop overt active disease months later.

Prognostic Factors

In patients who have limited chronic GVHD the prognosis is usually good; it is less favorable in those with untreated extensive disease. In addition, the type of onset of chronic GVHD has prognostic significance (Fig. 7): chronic GVHD which progresses from unresolved acute GVHD has an unfavorable prognosis. In contrast, patients with *de novo* chronic GVHD (i.e., no preceding acute GVHD) have the best prognosis, and those with "quiescent" onset (i.e., after complete resolution of acute GVHD) have an intermediate prognosis. Failure to respond to initial therapy is also a poor prognostic factor. Furthermore, patients with extensive chronic GVHD and persistent thrombocytopenia ($<100 \times 10^9$/L) have an increased mortality. The pathogenesis of thrombocytopenia is largely unknown, but is assumed to be related to the immuno-regulatory abnormalities in GVHD affecting the hematopoietic system. Most of these patients have hypocellular marrow aspirates. Lichenoid changes on skin histology and an elevated serum bilirubin have been identified as additional predictors of poor outcome; the latter is presumably a marker for the degree of bile-duct damage. About 70% of patients with none of those risk factors are expected to survive, as compared with about 50% with one risk factor and less than 20% with two or more of these risk factors.

Prophylaxis

Since acute GVHD represents a risk factor for the development of subsequent chronic GVHD, attempts to prevent chronic GVHD are aimed at reducing the incidence and severity of acute GVHD. Methotrexate and cyclosporine, either alone or in combination, are administered starting shortly before and shortly after marrow infusion and at regular intervals thereafter as prophylaxis against acute GVHD. Surprisingly, the incidence of chronic GVHD with this regimen has not been significantly reduced. Conversely, prevention of acute GVHD by T-cell depletion can also lower the incidence of chronic GVHD. Prolonged low-dose administration of glucocorticoids has been recommended by some as prophylaxis for chronic GVHD.

In patients with severe aplastic anemia the infusion of viable donor buffy coat cells can enhance the engraftment rate but is associated with a significantly higher incidence of chronic GVHD. However, most centers have abandoned this approach and have instead incorporated total body or total lymphoid irradiation or anti-thymocyte globulin into the conditioning regimen in order to achieve engraftment.

Specific Treatment

Patients who have limited chronic GVHD (Table 27) are usually not treated but are monitored closely to observe any progression of the disease. Patients with subclinical chronic GVHD (positive lip or skin biopsy only) should also not receive treatment, as higher rates of leukemic relapse have been observed in those receiving treatment, possibly due to a lack of graft-versus-leukemia effect (see below). These patients should be followed closely and treated as "standard-risk" patients when clinical symptoms develop. The natural course of extensive chronic GVHD is unfavorable and almost all such patients will have some degree of disability. There are a few anecdotal reports of untreated patients whose chronic GVHD "burned out" 5–10 years post-BMT. However, some of these patients are severely disabled from contractures, runting and occasionally blindness. Treatment must be instituted early in the course of chronic GVHD, since late therapy cannot influence the unfavorable course of the disease. In patients with "standard risk" chronic GVHD either daily cyclosporine or every second day prednisone is recommended. Since thalidomide has shown some effects in otherwise treatment-resistant chronic GVHD, it is now being studied in standard-risk patients. Side effects such as sleepiness and neuropathy can occur.

Patients who have extensive chronic GVHD along with persistent thrombocytopenia (platelets less than $100 \times 10^9/L$) or those who have failed initial therapy of chronic GVHD belong to a "high-risk" group and require more intensive treatment for a longer period of time. The combination of prednisone and cyclosporine has proven to be the most efficacious combination. The dosage schedule of the two drugs differs somewhat from center to center. The Seattle group introduced an alternate-day regimen giving 1 mg/kg/day prednisone on day A, and cyclosporine 6 mg/kg every 12 hours on day B. Because cyclosporine is stored in lipid tissue and released in a delayed fashion, it can still be found in serum on the "off day" in about half the patients. Side effects of the combination treatment with cyclosporine and prednisone (e.g., hypertension and renal insufficiency) are common, but most patients are able to continue treatment. Aseptic necrosis of the bone (most often the hip) occurs in about 5% of patients and usually requires discontinuation of the steroids. Modifications of this regimen are being utilized, such as the simultaneous administration of prednisone and cyclosporine for a few weeks as induction therapy and the subsequent administration of cyclosporine as maintenance. Other centers prefer to give cyclosporine as a single treatment and add corticosteroids when the disease flares. As a general guideline, patients should be treated for at least 9–12 months and then reassessed including biopsies (skin, lip).

A complete response is defined as normal skin and lip biopsies and no clinical or laboratory evidence of chronic GVHD. Treatment should then be tapered over 8–12 weeks. If there is no return of symptoms within 6 months after discontinuation of therapy, then these patients usually have developed stable graft-host tolerance. About 15–20% of all patients will have a flare of GVHD activity within the first 6 months after discontinuation of the immunosuppressive treatment and, depending on severity, it may be necessary to resume treatment. If there is no clinical GVHD but biopsies continue to be positive at the "1-year workup", then this partial response requires treatment for another 9–12 months. Some patients with drug-resistant chronic GVHD of the mouth or skin may benefit from a combination of psoralen and ultraviolet irradiation (PUVA). GVHD confined to the mouth can be treated with some success by mouth rinsing with corticosteroids (dexamethasone 0.25%). Resistant chronic GVHD may progress despite all therapeutic efforts, and new approaches to salvage therapy (e.g., FK506) are needed.

Supportive Care and Immunization

These measures are primarily aimed at preventing recurrent infection and disability. They include prophylactic antibiotics, oral hygiene, artificial saliva and tears, nutritional support and sun-blocking creams (protection factor ≥ 15). To prevent vaginal stenosis, topical estrogen creams as well as systemic estrogen/progesterone combinations are recommended. Female patients on long-term treatment with steroids should be an equal dose of Medoxyprogesteron to their dose of steroids. Also, calcium (1000 mg/day) and multivitamins (providing 400 IU of vitamin D) are recommended to prevent bone loss. To prevent esophageal disease, antacids, ranitidine and elevation of the head of the bed may be employed. The administration of intravenous gammaglobulins may be beneficial, especially in patients with IgG subclass deficiency. However because of the high cost of such treatment, further data as to the long-term effectiveness of passive immunotherapy are needed.

Infectious Complications with Chronic GVHD

Except for varizella zoster, the incidence of infections in long-term stable patients without chronic GVHD is not higher than in normal healthy people. However, the immunological disorders seen in patients with chronic GVHD predispose them to late infections, mostly with encapsulated bacteria and viruses. With control of GVHD, the incidence of these infections is usually reduced. Sinusitis, otitis media and upper respiratory system infections frequently due to encapsulated organisms (e.g., *S. pneumoniae*, *H. influenzae*) occur more frequently, in part secondary to a persistent IgG_2 subclass deficiency. Patients who develop chronic GVHD after an unrelated-donor transplant have an even higher incidence of bacteremia and/or septicemia.

There is still some uncertainty as to the best method of infection prophylaxis in these patients. Most patients will receive trimethoprim-sulfamethoxazole daily or at least twice weekly to protect them from infections with both *Pneumocystis carinii* and gram-positive organisms. If for some reason this drug cannot be given, penicillin is recommended instead. At some centers, ongoing studies are trying to answer the question of whether or not regular intravenous gammaglobulin application can effectively prevent infections in these patients. Patients with extensive chronic GVHD have been shown to have functional asplenia which can be documented by the presence of Howell-Jolly bodies on routine blood smears; spleen size is reduced in these patients. This asplenia is believed to contribute to an increased susceptibility to bacterial infections, and these patients may benefit from long-term antibiotic prophylaxis.

Chronic GVHD in Children

Chronic GVHD in children is less common than in adults, due to the fact that children less frequently develop acute GVHD. Symptoms and treatment options are similar to those in adults. However, children with chronic GVHD can have diminished height and height velocity as well as deficiencies in growth and thyroid hormone levels. The "hormonal balance" is further perturbed by long-term steroid treatment. It is of note that children may have an increased cyclosporine clearance, causing lower levels of the drug on standard doses.

Graft-Versus-Leukemia Effect

In 1956, Barnes observed that a transplanted marrow graft can destroy residual leukemic cells in lethally irradiated mice. This graft versus leukemia (GVL) effect can also be shown in patients who develop acute or chronic GVHD, and is further supported by the observation that patients with identical twin donors on average have a two-fold increase in relapse rate when compared to allogeneic recipients with the same disease. Analysis of clinical studies in patients after syngeneic, autologous and allogeneic bone marrow transplantation have shown that leukemia is not eradicated only by high-dose chemo- and radiotherapy – the immune mechanisms also play an important role. T-lymphocytes, natural killer cells or cytokines released in the course of acute or chronic GVHD may be the mediators of this effect.

Vaccination after Marrow Transplantation

Most investigators now agree that the majority of patients will require revaccination ≥12 months post-transplant. It is advisable to give the diphtheria/tetanus (DT) vaccine first and assess response (if available) 6–8 weeks later by measuring tetanus toxoid antibody levels. If the patient has responded to DT, 23 valent pneumoccocal vaccine, 14 valent meningococcal vaccine and *Hemophilus influenza* (HIB) protein conjugate vaccine should be administered. Booster vaccine for the polysaccharides antigens (pneumoccocal, meningococcal and HIB) is advised 12 months later (at about 24 months). Killed polio (Salk) vaccine should be given 1–2 years after BMT.

The use of live vaccines, specifically measles/mumps/rubella (MMR) should be limited to the study setting, in either autologous BMT patients or allogeneic BMT patients who are free of GVHD and off immunosuppression.

Persons in immediate contact with the marrow recipient should not receive oral live polio vaccine, but may receive MMR.

References

Atkinson K, Bryant D, Delprado W, Biggs J (1989) Widespread pulmonary fibrosis as a major clinical manifestation of chronic graft-versus-host disease. Bone Marrow Transplant 4:129

Atkinson K, Horowitz MM, Gale RP, Lee MB, Rimm AA, Bortin MM (1989) Consensus among bone marrow transplanters for diagnosis, grading and treatment of chronic graft-versus-host disease. Bone Marrow Transplant 4:247

Corson SL, Sullivan K, Batzer F, August C, Storb R, Thomas ED (1982) Gynecologic manifestations of chronic graft-versus-host disease. Obstet Gynecol 60:488

Ferrara JLM, Deeg HJ (1991) Graft-versus-host disease. N Engl J Med 324:667

Franklin RM, Kenyon KR, Tutschka PJ, Saral R, Green WR, Santos G (1983) Ocular manifestations of chronic graft-versus-host disease. Ophthalmology 90:4

Holland HK, Wingard JR, Beschorner WE, Saral R, Santos GW (1988) Bronchiolitis obliterans in bone marrow transplantation and its relationship to chronic graft-v-host disease and low serum IgG. Blood 72:621

Horowitz MM, Gale RP, Sondel PM, Goldman JM, Kersey J, Kolb H-J, Rimm AA, Ringden O, Rozman C, Speck B, Truitt RL, Zwaan FE, Bortin MM (1990) Graft-versus-leukemia reactions after bone marrow transplantation. Blood 75:555

Kalhs P, Panzer S, Kletter K, Minar E, Stain-Kos M, Walter R, Lechner K, Hinterberger W (1988) Functional asplenia after bone marrow transplantation: A late complication related to extensive chronic graft-versus-host disease. Ann Intern Med 109:461

Klingemann H-G, Phillips GL (1991) Immunotherapy after bone marrow transplantation. Bone Marrow Transplant 8:73

Loughran Jr TP, Sullivan K, Morton T, Beckham C, Schubert M, Witherspoon R, Sale G, Sanders J, Fisher L, Shulman H, Thomas ED, Storb R (1990) Value of day 100 screening studies for predicting the development of chronic graft-versus-host disease after allogeneic bone marrow transplantation. Blood 76:228

Lum LG (1987) The kinetics of immune reconstitution after human marrow transplantation. Blood 69:369

McDonald GB, Sullivan KM, Plumley TF (1984) Radiographic features of esophageal involvement in chronic graft-vs-host disease. AJR Am J Roentgenol 142:501

Rouquette-Gally AM, Boyeldieu D, Gluckman E, Abuaf N, Combrisson A (1987) Autoimmunity in 28 patients after allogeneic bone marrow transplantation: Comparison with Sjogren syndrome and scleroderma. Br J Haematol 66:45

Sale GE, Shulmann HM, Schubert MM, Sullivan KM, Kopecky KJ, Hackman RC, Morton TH, Storb R, Thomas ED (1981) Oral and ophthalmic pathology of graft-versus-host disease in man: Predictive value of the lip biopsy. Hum Pathol 12:1022

Schubert HM, Sullivan KM, Morton TH, Izutsu KT, Peterson DE, Flournoy N, Truelove EL, Sale GE, Buckner CD, Storb R, Thomas ED (1984) Oral manifestation of chronic graft versus host disease. Ann Intern Med 144:1591

Sheridan JF, Tutschka PJ, Sedmak DD, Copelan EA (1990) Immunoglobulin G subclass deficiency and pneumococcal infection after allogeneic bone marrow transplantation. Blood 75:1583

Shulman HM, Sullivan KM, Weiden PL, McDonald GB, Striker GE, Sale GE, Hackman RC, Tsoi MD, Storb R, Thomas ED (1980) Chronic graft-versus-host syndrome in man. A long-term clinicopathologic study of 20 Seattle patients. Am J Med 69:204

Sullivan KM, Shulman HM, Storb R, Weiden PL, Witherspoon RP, McDonald GB, Schubert MM, Atkinson K, Thomas ED (1981) Chronic graft-versus-host disease in 52 patients: Adverse natural course and successful treatment with combination immunosuppression. Blood 57:267

Sullivan KM, Witherspoon RP, Storb R, Deeg HJ, Dahlberg S, Sanders JE, Appelbaum FR, Doney KC, Weiden P, Anasetti C, Loughran TP, Hill R, Shields A, Yee G, Shulman H, Nims J, Strom S, Thomas ED (1988) Alternating-day cyclosporine and prednisone for treatment of high-risk chronic graft-v-host disease. Blood 72:555

Sullivan KM, Witherspoon RP, Storb R, Weiden P, Flournoy N, Dahlberg S, Deeg HJ, Sanders JE, Doney KC, Appelbaum FR, McGuffin R, McDonald GB, Meyers J, Schubert MM, Gauvreau J, Shulman HM, Sale GE, Anasetti C, Loughran TP, Strom S, Nims J, Thomas ED (1988) Prednisone and azathioprine compared with prednisone and placebo for treatment of chronic graft-v-host disease: Prognostic influence of prolonged thrombocytopenia after allogeneic marrow transplantation. Blood 72:546

Sullivan KM, Weiden PL, Storb R, Witherspoon RP, Fefer A, Fisher L, Buckner CD, Anasetti C, Appelbaum FR, Badger C, Beatty P, Bensinger W, Berenson R, Bigelow C, Cheever MA, Clift R, Deeg HJ, Doney K, Greenberg P, Hansen JA, Hill R, Loughran T, Martin P, Neiman P, Petersen FB, Sanders J, Singer J, Stewart P, Thomas ED (1989) Influence of acute and chronic graft-versus-host disease on relapse and survival after bone marrow transplantation from HLA-identical siblings as treatment of acute and chronic leukemia. Blood 73:1720

Tanaka K, Sullivan KM, Shulman HM, Sale GE, Tanaka A (1991) A clinical review: Cutaneous manifestations of acute and chronic graft-versus-host disease following bone marrow transplantation. J Dermatol 18:11

Weiden PL, Sullivan KM, Flournoy N, Storb R, Thomas ED (1981) Antileukemic effect of chronic graft-versus-host disease: Contribution to improved survival after allogeneic marrow transplantation. N Engl J Med 304:1529

Wingard JR, Piantadosi S, Vogelsang GB, Farmer ER, Jabs DA, Levin S, Beschorner WE, Cahill RA, Miller DF, Harrison D, Saral R, Santos GW (1989) Predictors of death from chronic graft-versus-host disease after bone marrow transplantation. Blood 74:1428

Wood PMD, Proctor SJ (1990) The potential use of thalidomide in the therapy of graft-versus-host disease – a review of clinical and laboratory information. Leuk Res 14:395

3. Pulmonary Problems

Interstitial Pneumonitis and Pulmonary Infections

Acute pulmonary toxicity early after transplantation is mainly related to high dose chemo/radiotherapy and manifests itself as interstitial pneumonitis (IP); there are also numerous infectious agents that can affect the lung early post-transplant. The majority of cases of IP occur within the first 3 months post BMT (see III.5). Late-onset IP is relatively uncommon, occurring in only about 5% of patients, and is usually caused by a heterogenous group of pathogens, mainly of an infectious nature. Patients who have chronic GVHD requiring immunosuppressive treatment are at risk for *Pneumocystis carinii* pneumonia. This group is also predominantly at risk for viral infections, which present clinically as interstitial pneumonitis. Common viruses are CMV, VZV and RSV.

The probability of infectious pulmonary complications decreases with time after transplant; however, in recipients who develop chronic GVHD, pulmonary infections can occur as a delayed and sometimes recurrent problem. These infections are presumably related to a decrease in the mucociliary clearance mechanism, immunoregulatory defects, and the reduced production of secretory IgA.

Restrictive Pulmonary Disease

Mild restrictive defects of ventilatory function are seen in about 20% of patients after transplantation with the most severe effect noted at 1 year. Even in otherwise-healthy long-term survivors, sequential pulmonary function studies have shown some loss of total lung capacity, a decrease in vital capacity, and mild impairment of diffusing capacity at 1 year after bone marrow transplantation in about 25% of patients. However, in one particular study, lung function improved over the subsequent 3 to 4 years. The restrictive pulmonary changes are apparently not correlated with any particular type of conditioning regimen or the presence of chronic GVHD, although it is known that chemotherapy can cause interstitial pulmonary changes with subsequent fibrosis and restrictive losses in function. Patients who have IP early in their post-transplant course tend to have greater restrictive changes subsequently. Generally these restrictive pulmonary changes do not produce severe symptoms and therefore do not require therapeutic intervention, but it is not clear whether or to what extent they ultimately contribute to obstructive pulmonary changes.

Obstructive Pulmonary Disease

In general, one has to distinguish between the moderate obstruction that can occur post-transplant in patients who have received chemo- and radiotherapy, and obstructive lung disease due to lymphocytic bronchitis and bronchiolitis obliterans, which can be recognized histologically and frequently occur in conjunction with chronic GVHD.

Lymphocytic Bronchitis

This disease is often seen in patients who have symptoms of extensive chronic GVHD, and the histological changes seen in the lung are believed to be GVHD-related. The proximal bronchial mucosa, submucosa and muscularis are infiltrated by small lymphocytes, leading to an associated loss of ciliae. Mucosal necrosis and submucosal gland necrosis contribute to the loss of mucociliary clearance. This loss of local immunity may facilitate recurrent infections. Symptoms of lymphocytic bronchitis include dry cough, dyspnea, and occasional wheezing.

Most of these patients also have oral mucositis, esophagitis, sinusitis and oral and ocular sicca syndrome or other symptoms related to chronic GVHD. Another frequent finding in these patients is a decreased serum and secretory IgA level, which may predispose to recurrent infections of the small airways which contribute to the development of chronic obstructive lung disease. Moreover, repeated aspiration caused by esophageal abnormalities related to chronic GVHD may also contribute to the pathogenesis of obstructive lung disease. Similarly, sinusitis is a frequent problem after transplantation, and the aspiration of purulent sinus secretions may contribute to the development of chronic obstructive airway disease. Therefore, patients with symptoms of chronic pulmonary problems, such as cough, wheezing, and dyspnea on exertion, should undergo the following studies:

- Pulmonary function tests
- Sinus and esophageal radiography
- Determination of serum immunoglobulin levels
- Tests to evaluate the activity of chronic GVHD

Early treatment of the underlying disorder may prevent the development of progressive obstructive lung disease.

Bronchiolitis Obliterans

Progressive bronchiolitis obliterans has also been linked to chronic GVHD. Bronchiolitis obliterans affects about 10% of all patients who have active chronic GVHD, and its clinical course can vary from mild and slow progression to diffuse necrotizing bronchiolitis of the small airways leading to death of the patient. Unexplained cough is often the presenting symptom, with dyspnea in more severe cases. Histologically one can see an acute exudative bronchiolitis forming intraluminal plugs containing mononuclear cells and necrotic epithelium in a matrix or proteinaceous exudate rich in fibrin (Fig. 12). Later organization may lead to mature mucopolysaccharide rich connective tissue with fibroblasts. The clinical correlate is known as bronchiolitis obliterans organizing pneumonia (BOOP). Additional risk factors for the development of bronchiolitis obliterans include transplants from HLA-nonidentical donors and immunosuppressive therapy with

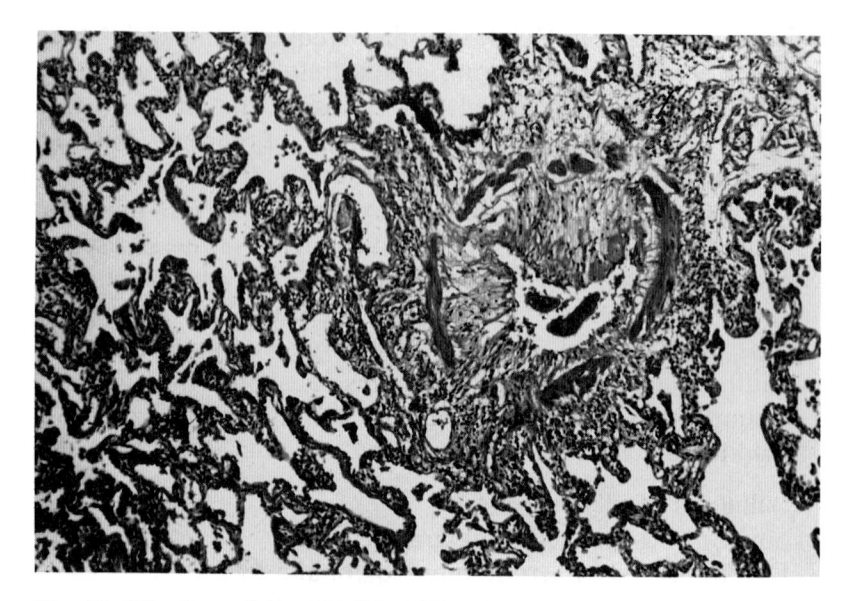

Fig. 12. Histology of bronchiolitis obliterans. Lung tissue showing fibrous obliteration of one bronchiole

methotrexate. In some cases bronchiolitis obliterans appears to be precipitated by viral (e.g., RSV, parainfluenza III) or bacterial infections. Bronchiolitis obliterans is not seen after autotransplants, and there is no association with any particular preparative regimen or prior history of respiratory illness. It is presumed that low serum and secretory immunoglobulin levels and sinubronchial sicca could predispose to bronchiolitis obliterans via airway colonization, irritation and obstruction. Chest films may show hyperinflation of the lungs and flattening of the diaphragm, but are often not diagnostic. Recurrent pneumothoraces have been reported. Pulmonary function tests can show an obstructive pattern with a marked reduction in forced midexpiratory flow to 10–20% of predicted values, and moderate to severe reduction in FEV_1/FVC.* These changes indicate airflow obstruction, especially involving small airways, which is not responsive to bronchodilators. In contrast, the carbon monoxide transfer coefficient is normal in these patients, suggesting good gas exchange in the lung tissue.

---

*FEV_1 = Forced expiratory volume in 1 second; FVC = Forced vital capacity

Bronchiolitis obliterans has been observed as early as several months after marrow transplantation, and the majority of patients who develop the complication do so within 2 years after marrow grafting. It is not clear at present whether bronchiolitis obliterans is a primary manifestation of chronic GVHD or whether mucociliary changes associated with long-standing chronic GVHD merely facilitate its development. In progressive cases treatment options are limited, and characteristically this disease does not respond to therapy with bronchodilators. Prompt treatment of infections as well as appropriate therapy of chronic GVHD seem to be of benefit in this disease. The role of immunoglobulin replacement in patients with low serum IgG and IgA levels is unclear, but such treatment is generally recommended to prevent bronchiolitis obliterans in predisposed patients. Some centers give a 14-day course of high dose steroids (10 mg/kg) to get the disease under control and then maintain control with established chronic GVHD treatment protocols such as the combination of cyclosporine and prednisone. It appears that outcome is worse in patients with early onset and greater reduction in FEV_1. The differential diagnosis of bronchiolitis obliterans includes asthma that can be pre-existing in the recipient or acquired from the donor via transferred immune response. Classical asthma, in contrast to bronchiolitis obliterans, will respond well to treatment with bronchodilators.

Pulmonary Vascular Abnormalities

Pulmonary Embolism

Pulmonary thrombi/emboli have been found at autopsy in up to 50% of patients after allogeneic bone marrow transplantation. Although their etiology is not clear, it may be that the infusion of even filtered bone marrow can cause some degree of thrombosis in pulmonary vessels. These emboli are usually scattered and demonstrated only in arterioles, capillaries and venules. Usually there are no signs of muscular hyperplasia or intimal thickening. It is difficult to assess whether these pulmonary emboli can contribute to any post-transplant abnormalities in pulmonary function such as decrease in diffusing capacity.

Veno-Occlusive Disease

Patients who have received BCNU as part of their preparative regimen may present with a rather sudden-onset IP occurring usually between 2–4 months after BMT. Clinically these patients present with arterial hypoxemia and pulmonary hypertension. Histologic changes of venoocclusive disease with partial to complete occlusion of pulmonary veins and venules by loose fibrous proliferation of the intima may be seen. High-dose steroid treatment can stop progression of the disease and may lead to resolution.

References

Beschorner WE, Saral R, Hutchings GM (1978) Lymphocytic bronchitis associated with graft-versus-host disease in recipients of bone marrow transplants. N Engl J Med 299:1030

Chan CK, Hyland RH, Hutcheon MA, Minden MD, Alexander MA, Kossakowska AE (1987) Small airways disease in recipients of allogeneic bone marrow transplant. Medicine (Baltimore) 66:324

Clark JG, Crawford SW, Madtes DK, Sullivan KM (1989) Obstructive lung disease after allogeneic marrow transplantation: Clinical presentation and course. Ann Intern Med 111:368

Clark JG, Schwartz DA, Flournoy N, Sullivan KM, Crawford SW, Thomas ED (1987) Risk factors for airflow obstruction in recipients of bone marrow transplants. Ann Intern Med 107:648

Hackman RC, Madtes DK, Petersen FB, Clark JG (1989) Pulmonary venoocclusive disease following bone marrow transplantation. Transplantation 47:989

Holland HK, Wingard JR, Beschorner WE, Saral R, Santos GW (1988) Bronchiolitis obliterans in bone marrow transplantation and its relationship to chronic graft-v-host disease and low serum IgG. Blood 72:621

Prince DS, Wingard JR, Saral R, Santos GW, Wise RA (1989) Longitudinal changes in pulmonary function following bone marrow transplantation. Chest 96:301

Ralph DD, Springmeyer SC, Sullivan KM, Hackman RC, Storb R, Thomas ED (1984) Rapidly progressive airflow obstruction in marrow transplant recipients: Possible association between obliterative bronchiolitis and chronic graft-versus-host disease. Am Rev Respir Dis 129:641

Springmeyer SC, Silvestri RC, Flournoy N, Kosanke CW, Peterson DL, Huseby JS, Hudson LD, Storb R, Thomas ED (1984) Pulmonary function of marrow transplant patients. I. Effects of marrow infusion, acute graft-versus-host disease, and interstitial pneumonitis. Exp Hematol 12:805

Wingard JR, Santos GW, Saral R (1985) Late-onset interstitial pneumonia following allogeneic bone marrow transplantation. Transplantation 39:21

4. Neuroendocrine Function, Growth and Development

Radiochemotherapy affects not only the intended target cells and tissues, i.e., lymphohemopoietic cells and tumor cells, but the entire organism. The most important factor is radiation. Current knowledge suggests that adverse effects are fewer, less severe or shorter lasting in patients conditioned with chemotherapy alone.

Thyroid Function

Studies at several marrow transplant centers have shown that while children conditioned with chemotherapy only generally have normal thyroid function, thyroid dysfunction is frequent in those conditioned with radiation-containing regimens. Thyroid dysfunction was diagnosed as early as one, and as late as 15 years after transplantation. Among patients given 10 Gy single dose TBI, 30–55% had compensated hypothyroidism (with normal T4 and elevated TSH), and 10–15% had overt hypothyroidism. In patients given fractionated TBI, 10–20% had compensated and approximately 3% had overt hypothyroidism. The incidence was somewhat lower in adult than in pediatric patients. Since untreated compensated hypothyroidism has been suggested as a factor in the development of neoplastic thyroid disease, it is advisable to treat these patients with thyroid supplementation, and re-evaluate them sequentially for many years following transplantation.

In addition to hypothyroidism there have been some reports of hyperthyroidism, generally in patients with chronic GVHD.

Adrenal Glands

Only limited data on adrenal gland dysfunction following transplantation are available. Sanders and colleagues found that 24% of 78 patients examined from 1–8 years after transplant (while not on glucocorticoid treatment) had subnormal 11-desoxycortisol levels. None of these patients was symptomatic, and the percentage of patients developing abnormalities appeared to remain relatively constant with time after transplant. Although this study did not differentiate between primary and secondary adrenal insufficiency, the finding of subnormal stimulated cortisol levels is similar to that reported in patients given central nervous system irradiation. Further studies are necessary to determine whether these patients are able to handle physiological stress in a normal fashion.

Growth

Sanders and colleagues have shown that both male and female pediatric patients prepared for transplantation with TBI containing regimens have depressed growth velocity curves and do not experience a growth spurt in early adolescence. Growth velocity was further dampened in patients who also suffered from chronic GVHD. This change in growth velocity did not appear to be dependent upon treatment of chronic GVHD with glucocorticoids. No catch-up growth was observed after discontinuing treatment for chronic GVHD. Furthermore the lag in age adjusted growth did not decrease with increasing time after transplantation. Growth impairment was more severe with single dose TBI than with fractionated TBI, and in patients given previous cranial irradiation than in those without cranial irradiation. Among children who had received cranial irradiation and were prepared with TBI, 87% had subnormal growth hormone levels; without prior cranial irradiation the incidence was 42%. Furthermore, the younger the patient at the time of irradiation and the higher the dose of TBI, the more severe was growth retardation. However, growth is affected by factors other than growth hormone. The fact that the type of TBI (single dose vs. fractionated) did not affect growth until approximately three years following transplant suggests that fractionated TBI allows for some repair and recovery, albeit delayed, of epiphyseal, metaphyseal, and diaphyseal bone growth. For the majority of patients radiological bone age was within two years of the chronologic age. Only a small fraction of patients lagged behind more than 2 years, and half of those had chronic GVHD which generally had been treated with glucocorticoids.

The fact that children do not show growth acceleration after discontinuing treatment with glucocorticoids has led to speculation that somatomedin may be abnormal (due to impaired synthesis in the liver), and thus, may contribute to abnormal growth rates. No studies on replacement have been reported. It is also conceivable that abnormal gonadal and thyroid hormone levels play a role in this multifactorial growth abnormality. It will, furthermore, be of interest to determine whether children treated for GVHD without glucocorticoids, for example with cyclosporine, show improved linear growth rates. The administration of growth hormone has met with only limited success.

Sexual Development

Sanders et al. Studied girls and boys, 1–13 years of age at the time of transplantation. The majority of children prepared with 10 Gy single exposure TBI showed delayed development and slow progression of secondary sexual characteristics due to primary (hypergonadotropic) hypogonadism.

In girls the development of breast stage and pubic hair according to the criteria of Tanner and Whitehouse was delayed in virtually all instances, and some had delayed menarche. All girls who were past puberty at the time of transplantation remained amenorrheic with elevated LH and FSH levels, and decreased estradiol levels for at least 3–14 years; eventually, some of these women have shown recovery of ovarian function with hormonal levels returning toward normal. Among 4 women who had spontaneous menses 3–5 years after transplantation, one became pregnant and had an elective abortion. In order to avoid symptoms of menopause, cyclic hormone supplementation should be offered.

Similarly, boys had delayed pubertal development of penis and pubic hair stage, as well as testicular volume. Many boys had normal LH levels associated with normal FSH and testosterone levels, and these showed higher developmental scores than those with normal levels. Semen analysis showed azoospermia.

In patients conditioned with regimens not containing TBI there was only very mild derangement of growth and sexual development. Within months of transplantation vertical growth resumed and patients reached normal or close to normal height. There was a mild delay in sexual maturation, but unless interfered with by severe chronic GVHD, development was normal.

Fertility

All women who are post-pubertal at the time of transplantation appear to become amenorrheic for some time post-transplant. These women generally have symptoms of menopause and require hormone replacement. In one study, less than 5% recovered ovarian function, 3 to 7 years after transplantation, but at least 5 women have become pregnant and one has delivered a normal child.

In women conditioned only with chemotherapy, generally cyclophosphamide, the outcome is strongly dependent upon age at the time of transplantation. In one study patients less than 26 years of age recovered ovarian function 3 to 42 months after transplant, whereas about two thirds of women 26 years of age or older developed primary ovarian failure. At least 15 women who regained ovarian function have become pregnant, and 21 normal children were born.

Results are somewhat different in men. Among patients given TBI and chemotherapy more than 90% are found to be azoospermic, and 70–80% have elevated follicle stimulating hormone levels. However, almost 90% of patients have normal luteinizing hormone levels, and frequently normal plasma testosterone. One man with a return of sperm production has fathered three normal children.

In contrast, more men conditioned with chemotherapy only, generally cyclophosphamide, have a return of Sertoli cell function and sperm production and a normalization of follicle stimulating hormone, and usually also luteinizing hormone levels. Twenty-one men are known to have fathered twenty-eight normal children.

Thus, among adults the impact of the conditioning regimen used for marrow transplantation is less severe than in the pediatric population, but nevertheless is significant in regards to gonadal function. In women with iatrogenic menopause, hormone supplementation to prevent secondary complications of menopause such as vaginitis or osteoporosis is recommended.

References

Sanders JE (1990) Late effects in children receiving total body irradiation for bone marrow transplantation. Radiother Oncol 18(Suppl. 1):82–87

Sanders JE, Buckner CD, Sullivan KM, Doney K, Appelbaum F, Witherspoon R, Anasetti C, Storb R, Thomas ED. Growth and development after bone marrow transplantation. In: Buckner CD, Gale RP, Lucarelli G (eds), Advances and Controversies in Thalassemia Therapy: Bone Marrow Transplantation and Other Approaches. Alan R. Liss, New York; 375–382

Sanders JE, Buckner CD, Amos D, Levy W, Appelbaum FR, Doney K, Storb R, Sullivan KM, Witherspoon RP, Thomas ED (1988) Ovarian function following marrow transplantation for aplastic anemia or leukemia. J Clin Oncol 6:813–818

Sanders JE, Buckner CD, Leonard JM, Sullivan KM, Witherspoon RP, Deeg HJ, Storb R, Thomas ED (1983) Late effects on gonadal function of cyclophosphamide, total-body irradiation, and marrow transplantation. Transplantation 36:252–255

Sklar CA, Kim TH, Ramsay NKC (1982) Thyroid dysfunction among long-term survivors of bone marrow transplantation. Am J Med 73:688–694

Sklar CA, Kim TH, Ramsay NKC (1984) Testicular function following bone marrow transplantation performed during or after puberty. Cancer 53:1498–1501

Urban C, Schwingshandl J, Slavc I, Gamillscheg A, Hauer C, Schmid G, Kaulfersch W, Borkenstein M (1988) Endocrine function after bone marrow transplantation without the use of preparative total body irradiation. Bone Marrow Transplantation 3:291–296

5. Ophthalmologic Problems

During and following marrow transplantation the eye can be damaged in many ways. The conjunctivae are affected by chemotherapeutic agents and by viruses, the lacrimal glands can be involved by chronic GVHD or may show reduced tear production due to chemo-radiotherapy induced damage. There may be retinal hemorrhage and choroiditis. In addition, there are longterm effects, mostly affecting the lens.

It is known that irradiation can damage the ocular lens and lead to cataracts. This has been shown in patients undergoing localized irradiation to fields including the eyes, and in survivors of the atomic bomb explosions in Japan. Thus, it was expected that patients given TBI in preparation for marrow transplantation would also develop cataracts. We reported a study on 277 patients followed for 1–12 years. These patients had been prepared either with chemotherapy alone, or with TBI in combination with chemotherapy, with TBI being given as a single exposure or fractionated. Single dose TBI consisted of 10 Gy, fractionate TBI ranged from 12–15 Gy given over 6–7 days. While approximately 80% of patients given single does TBI developed cataracts over a course of 5–6 years following transplantation, only 20% of patients given fractionated TBI did so. The incidence with fractionated TBI was, in fact, identical to that observed with chemotherapy regimens only, and was thought to be related at least in part to concurrent treatment with glucocorticoid.

All cataracts involved the posterior capsule of the lens. Further analysis showed that the risk of developing cataracts was highest about 3 years after transplant, and subsequently declined. It was also of note that patients developing cataracts after single dose TBI were more symptomatic than those developing cataracts with fractionated TBI or with chemotherapy only. At least 50% of patients who developed cataracts after single dose TBI required surgical intervention within 2–6 years following transplant, compared to only 20% of patients given fractionate TBI and none of the patients given chemotherapy only. The risk for developing cataracts was somewhat higher in patients with acute lymphoblastic leukemia and chronic myelogenous leukemia than in patients with acute myeloid leukemias. The reason for this was not clear. However, it is conceivable that prior use of steroids, cranial irradiation, or busulfan might be predisposing factors.

A recent update involving a larger number of patients (M. Benyunes, unpublished observations) confirms the earlier analysis: the incidence of cataracts was 80% with single dose TBI, 50% with fractionated TBI >12 Gy, 34% with fractionated TBI <12 Gy, and 19% with chemotherapy.

Cataracts after marrow transplantation can be treated as in any other patient if no chronic GVHD of the eye exists. Treatment consists of implantation of intraocular lenses, or if for some reason this is not feasible, the use of contact lenses. In patients who have chronic GVHD and suffer from sicca syndrome of the eyes, one may want to delay intervention; the use of contact lenses should be avoided. In this setting, the only solution would be cataract glasses which is not satisfactory. Every effort should be made to improve the patient's condition so that a lens can be implanted.

Irradiation to the eyes has also been reported to cause retinopathy within 1–3 years following exposure. Findings included vascular occlusions, hemorrhages, micoraneurysms, neovascularization, retinal detachments, and optic nerve atrophy. These patients had generally been given 4000–5000 cGy or even higher doses to the eye. Although certain "nonspecific" ocular changes including retinal, have been observed after TBI and marrow transplantation, the doses used (920–1575 cGy) were in a range where radiation retinopathy would not be expected.

Other ocular problems generally appear to be related to chronic GVHD. These include ectropion, corneal stippling, ulceration or even perforation of the cornea, and occlusion of the naso-lacrimal duct.

References

Deeg HJ, Flournoy N, Sullivan KM, Sheehan K, Buckner CD, Sanders JE, Storb R, Witherspoon RP, Thomas ED (1984) Cataracts after total body irradiation and marrow transplantation: A sparing effect of dose fractionation. Int J Radiat Oncol Biol Phys 10:957–964

Franklin RM, Kenyon KR, Tutschka PJ, Saral R, Green WR, Santos, GW (1983) Ocular manifestations of graft-versus-host disease. Ophthamology 90:4

Hanada R, Ueoka Y (1989) Obstruction of nasolacrimal ducts closely related to graft-versus-host disease after bone marrow transplantation. Bone Marrow Transplant 4:125–126

Jack MK, Jack GM, Sale GE, Shulman HM, Sullivan KM (1983) Ocular manifestations of graft-v-host disease. Arch Ophthalmol 101:1080–1084

6. Secondary Malignancies

As marrow transplantation has been used more frequently and with greater success, the number of long-term survivors has grown steadily. As a result, the probability of detecting delayed side effects has increased. As described above, patients are usually prepared for transplantation with high doses of immunosuppressive/cytotoxic agents and irradiation, in the form of TBI or total lymphoid irradiation, given either alone or in combination. Following the transplant procedure, patients are profoundly immunoincompetent. In addition, most of them receive immunosuppressive drugs such as methotrexate, cyclosporine, methylprednisolone and others to prevent or treat GVHD. Cytotoxic agents, ionizing irradiation, and the use of immunosuppressive drugs are associated with an increased risk of developing malignancies. Malignant tumors have been observed in patients given immunosuppressive treatment after renal or cardiac transplantation. Furthermore, allogeneic interactions between donor and host cells may result in chronic antigenic stimulation and proliferation, particularly in patients with chronic GVHD. Consequently, there has been concern about an increased risk of secondary malignancies after marrow transplantation. Studies in dogs and rhesus monkeys given allogeneic or autologous marrow grafts have, indeed, shown an increased incidence of malignant tumors as compared to control animals.

We have recently reviewed the experience at our Center. Four groups of malignancies can be differentiated: leukemia in donor cells; host-cell derived leukemia different from the original disease; lymphoproliferative disorders; solid tumors (Table 30).

The occurrence of leukemia in donor cells was first reported in 1971. The pathogenesis is not clear; several hypotheses have

Table 30. Secondary malignancies

Recurrence of leukemia in donor-derived cells
Leukemia in host cells of lineage different from original disease
Lymphoproliferative disorders (donor > host origin)
– EBV positive
– EBV negative
Solid tumors (host origin)
– Adenocarcinoma
– Squamous cell carcinoma
– Basal cell carcinoma
– Glioblastoma multiforme
– Malignant melanoma
– Sarcoma

---

been proposed. Conceivably, donor lymphoid cells undergo transformation due to antigenic stimulation by host tissue as observed in mouse models of marrow transplantation. This appears less likely in man. If this were the case, one would expect similar events in many more human patients undergoing marrow transplantation. However, so far secondary malignancies have been observed predominantly (although not exclusively) in patients who were conditioned with regimens including the use of TBI. Alternatively, the host milieu in which the original leukemia had arisen might predispose to abnormal lymphohemopoietic maturation and proliferation of donor derived cells. It has also been suggested that normal cells might undergo fusion with residual host leukemia cells, and, following diploidization, give rise to new malignancies. Finally, an etiologic agent such as an oncogene or a virus present in host cells may be transferred (transfected) to donor cells. Initial reports suggested that recurrences in donor cells usually presented very early after transplantation, but cases have now been observed as late as six years after transplant. Preliminary analyses suggest that recurrences may be in donor derived cells in approximately 5% of the observed cases. With the application of molecular biology techniques such as restriction fragment length polymorphism analysis to clinical medicine, a clearer picture should emerge in the near future.

More recently some patients have been observed to develop a host-cell derived leukemia different from their original disease. Similar events have been observed in non-transplant patients; for example, acute myelogenous leukemia developed in children previously treated with epipodophyllotoxins for acute lymphoblastic leukemia. Conceivably, the transplant conditioning regimen or chemotherapy given before transplantation induced mutations in host cells which then survived beyond transplant and evolved clonally into a new leukemia.

Lymphoproliferative disorders different from the original disease usually develop within a few months to one year of transplantation. Histologically, these are most frequently pleomorphic B cell lymphomas. There is evidence that they arise from polyclonal proliferation which evolves into monoclonal proliferation. However, other histologies have been observed also. In most instances the lymphomas observed developed in cells of donor origin, and in many cases Epstein-Barr virus genomic sequences were identified in the cells.

The development of these lymphoproliferative disorders is more frequent in patients given very aggressive immunosuppressive therapy, especially for the treatment of GVHD. Agents used include antithymocyte globulin, monoclonal antibodies (anti-CD3), and cyclosporine. Lymphoproliferative disorders have also been observed in patients given marrow that had been depleted of T cells in vitro (using monoclonal antibodies and complement), and seem to be particularly frequent in patients given HLA nonidentical T cell depleted marrow. Presumably, the removal of T cells results in lack of regulation or in dysregulation of B lymphocytes. Present experience suggests that a more judicious use of immunosuppressive agents and a reduction in dose wherever possible may reduce the probability of such a malignancy developing.

Solid tumors develop with a greater delay after transplantation, with intervals to occurrence ranging from 1 to more than 15 years. Glioblastoma multiform, adenocarcinoma, squanomous cell carcinoma, basal cell carcinoma, malignant melanoma, and sarcomas have all been observed. Irradiation is suspected to be an important etiologic factor. This notion is further supported by a recent report projecting a 22% 10-year incidence of solid tumors in patients with severe aplastic anemia conditioned with cyclophosphamide and thoracoabdominal irradiation. This compares to an incidence of approximately 6% in similar patients prepared with cyclophosphamide only.

Superimposed may be an effect of chronic GVHD, the presence of continued (autoimmune) antigenic stimulation, and the treatment of GVHD with steroids or cytotoxic agents. It is of note, however, that recent preliminary analyses show that secondary malignancies develop also in patients given autologous transplants.

Although the occurrence of secondary malignancies is of concern, several factors should be considered: first, most of these patients were initially treated for a potentially fatal illness, and without the use of marrow transplantation many would have died within weeks or months. Second, malignant neoplasms have also been observed in nontransplant patients receiving chemotherapy only, or irradiation and chemotherapy without marrow transplantation. Third, it is conceivable that the development of a second neoplasm is favored by an underlying genetic defect, which had already led to the development of the initial hematologic malignancy. Further studies are needed to define the magnitude of this problem and to develop new approaches that may prevent this complication.

References

Boyd CN, Ramberg RE, Thomas ED (1982) The incidence of recurrence of leukemia in donor cells after allogeneic bone marrow transplantation. Leuk Res 6:833–837

Chalmers JL (1991) Epstein-Barr Virus lymphoproliferative disease associated with acquired immunodeficiency. Medicine 70:137–160

Deeg HJ, Witherspoon RP. Risk factors for the development of secondary malignancies after marrow transplantation. Hematol Oncol Clin North Am (in press)

Feig SA, Dreazen O, Simon M, Wiley F, Schreck R, Gale RP (1988) B cell acute lymphoblastic leukaemia (ALL) in donor cells following bone marrow transplantation for T cell ALL. Bone Marrow Transplantation 3:331–337

Fisher A, Blanche S, Le Bidois J, Bordigoni P, Garnier JL, Niaudet P, Morinet F, Le Deist F, Fisher AM, Criscelli C, Hirn M (1991) Anti B cell monoclonal antibodies in the treatment of severe B cell lymphoproliferative syndrome following bone marrow and organ transplantation. N Engl J Med 324:1451–1456

Lishner M, Paterson B, Kandel R, Fyles G, Curtis JE, Meharchand J, Minden MD, Messner HA (1990) Cutaneous and mucosal neoplasms in bone marrow transplant recipients. Cancer 65:473–476

Schmitz N, Johannson W, Schmidt G, Von der Helm R, Löeffer H (1987) Recurrence of acute lymphoblastic leukaemia in donor cells after allogeneic marrow transplantation associated with a deletion of the long art of chromosome 6. Blood 70:1099–1104

Shapiro RS, McClain K, Frizzera G, Gajl-Peczalska KJ, Kersey JH, Blazar BR, Arthur DC, Patton DF, Greenberg JS, Burke B, Ramsay NKC, McGlave P, Filipovich AH (1988) Epstein-Barr virus associated B cell lymphoproliferative disorders following bone marrow transplantation. Blood 71:1234–1243

Skinner JC, Gilbert EF, Hong R, Bozdech MJ, Flynn B, Borcherding W, Hafez GR, Arya S, Trigg ME, Finlay JL, Sondel PM (1988) B cell lymphoproliferative disorders following T cell depleted allogeneic bone marrow transplantation. Am J Pedia Hema Onc 10:112–119

Socie G, Henry-Amar M, Cosset JM, Devergie A, Girinsky T, Gluckman E (1991) Increased incidence of solid malignant tumors after bone marrow transplantation for severe aplastic anemia. Blood 78:277–279 (Abstract)

Witherspoon RP, Fisher LD, Schoch G, Martin P, Sullivan KM, Sanders J, Deeg HJ, Doney K, Thomas D, Storb R, Thomas ED (1989) Secondary cancers after bone marrow transplantation for leukemia or aplastic anemia. N Engl J Med 321:784–789

Zutter MM, Durnam DM, Hackman RC, Loughran TP, Jr., Kidd PG, Ashley RL, Petersdorf EW, Martin PJ, Thomas ED (1990) Secondary T-cell lymphoproliferation after marrow transplantation. Am J Clin Pathol 94:714–721

7. Other Delayed Complications

Conditioning regimens used for marrow transplantation, chronic GVHD and its treatment affect all organs, and side effects in addition to those classically recognized must be expected.

Dental Abnormalities

Irradiation to growing skeletal bones interferes with normal longitudinal growth (see above). Irradiation also affects facial bones and dental development. Dental abnormalities have been observed in children given localized irradiation for lymphoma or solid tumors; similar effects are seen in children given 10 cGy or more of TBI. These include blunting of the roots, incomplete calcification, premature apical closure, developmental arrest, enamel hypoplasia and microdontia. There can also be abnormal occlusion, hypoblastic mandible and micrognathia. Children less than 7 years of age at transplantation are most severely affected.

Aseptic Necrosis

Aseptic necrosis, especially of humerus and femur heads, is a well documented side effect of glucocorticoid therapy, and has also been observed after marrow transplantation, predominantly in patients with chronic GVHD. It is important to note, however, that aseptic necrosis can also occur after only short courses of high dose steroid therapy for acute GVHD, and can present with a marked delay after treatment. Numerous patients have required prosthetic joint replacement.

Genitourinary Dysfunction

Hemorrhagic cystitis after cyclophosphamide and busulfan treatment usually develops acutely; however, scarring and bladder shrinkage can lead to chronic urinary problems. Hemolytic uremic syndrome or thrombocytopenic purpura with renal failure have been observed with prolonged cyclosporine therapy or even after discontinuation of treatment.

Radiation nephritis has been described in autologous transplant recipients treated with aggressive combination chemotherapy prior to transplantation. Finally, recent case reports describe a delayed-onset nephrotic syndrome as a possible manifestation of chronic GVHD.

Atrophic vaginitis or vaginal stenosis may develop secondary to hormone deficiency or GVHD (see above).

Central Nervous System (CNS) and Intellectual Dysfunction

CNS defects have been described after intrathecal chemotherapy and cranial irradiation. Structural defects include white matter hypodensity, calcifications and ventricular dilatation. The latter has been correlated with memory loss, impairment in verbal fluency and hypothalamic-pituitary dysfunction.

More refined studies in children after marrow transplantation are only now being conducted. However, neuropsychological deficits are well recognized in children who have received long-term treatment for acute leukemia. Cranial irradiation is considered the most likely causative agent, and the effect seems to be inversely related to age. Preliminary studies in marrow transplant recipients yield similar results, indicating impaired cognitive functions and IQ scores that may be lower than in controls. Adult patients often complain of difficulties concentrating and short attention span.

References

Altmaier EM, Gingrich RD, Fyfe MA (1991) Two-year adjustment of bone marrow transplant survivors. Bone Marrow Transplant 7:311–316

Dahllöf G, Barr M, Bolme P, Modeer T, Lönnqvist B, Ringden O, Heimdahl A (1988) Disturbances in dental development after total body irradiation in bone marrow transplant recipients. Oral Surg Oral Med Oral Pathol 65:41–44

Dahllöf G, Forsberg CM, Ringden O, Bolme P, Borgstrom B, Nasman M, Heimdahl A, Modeer T. Facial growth and morphology in long-term survivors after bone marrow transplantation. Eur J Orthod (in press)

Gomez-Garcia P, Herrara-Arroyo C, Torrez-Gomez A, et al. (1988) Renal involvement in chronic graft-versus-host disease: A report of two cases. Bone Marrow Transplant 3:357–362

Hiess EC, Goldschmidt E, Santelli G, et al. (1988) Membranous neophropathy in a bone marrow transplant recipient. Am J Kidney Dis 11:188–191

Juckett M, Perry EH, Daniels BS, Weisdorf DJ (1991) Hemolytic uremic syndrome following bone marrow transplantation. Bone Marrow Transplant 7:405–409

McGuire T, Sanders JE, Hill D, Buckner CD, Sullivan KM (1991) Neuropsychological function in children given total body irradiation for marrow transplantation. Exp Hematol 19:578 (Abstract)

Schubert MM, Sullivan KM, Truelove EL (1986) Head and neck complications of bone marrow transplantation, Chap. 21. In: Peterson ED, Sonis ST, Elias EG (eds), Head and Neck Management of the Cancer Patient. Martinus Nijhoff, Boston 401–427

Schubert MA, Sullivan KM, Schubert MM, Nims J, Hansen M, Sanders JE, O'Quigley J, Witherspoon RP, Buckner CD, Storb R, Thomas ED (1990) Gynecological abnormalities following allogeneic bone marrow transplantation. Bone Marrow Transplantation 5:425–430

Tarbell NJ, Guinan EC, Niemeyer C, et al. (1988) Late onset of renal dysfunction in survivors of bone marrow transplantation. Int J Rad Oncol Biol PHys 15:99–104

8. Rehabilitation

Research on issues of survivorship in cancer patients in general and marrow transplant patients in particular has begun only recently, and information is limited. Survival is a rather generic concept and includes everyone regardless of the disease course. However, long term adjustments and rehabilitation depend strongly upon events along the way.

The acute survival period, maybe the first year after transplantation, often is of great emotional intensity and dominated by fear. Complications are usually due to the conditioning regimen, poor engraftment, impaired immunocompetence and GVHD. In some patients disease recurrence is the overwhelming factor.

In patients with chronic GVHD changes in body image may be the most significant factor, due to skin disfigurement, malaise and weight loss. Medications, especially glucocorticoids may cause alterations of mood, and physical manifestations such as cushingoid features, weakness, osteoporosis and aseptic necrosis may be prominent. Cyclosporine may cause hirsutism and tremor.

Since treatment is often prolonged and complex, compliance may be poor. This in turn may worsen the symptoms and findings which may further undermine confidence and long term outlook. Along with fear of disease recurrence this may lead to severe depression which can be worsened by fatigue, changes in partner relationships and family roles. Patients may consider themselves, and in fact be, a burden to the family. Patients may change their life priorities and perspectives, and accepting these changes is often difficult for those around them. As the interval from transplantation grows, adjusting to home, school and work situations becomes more important. The ability to do so depends upon an individual's coping skills.

Patients without chronic GVHD, chronic pulmonary problems or sequelae of treatment (e.g., aseptic necrosis) tend to move towards normal activities within a year or two of transplantation. The role of the medical team diminishes and patients and families are at times struggling to refind their places in the "real" world.

As patients continue to worry about the possibility of recurrence of their disease, planning for the future becomes a difficult task. Considerable adjustments in life style and profession may be required for those who have suffered sequelae such as cataracts, skin contractures and muscle wasting. Among adolescents, issues with sexuality or sexual maturation arise frequently, sooner or later after transplantation. The healthy partner, after long periods of stress an deprivation, may put demands on the transplant patient which he or she may not be able or willing to fulfill. This may further contribute to intramarital stress and, along with social and financial demands, may result in marital dysfunction and divorce.

Problems with employment and insurance may occur, and discrimination is not infrequent. Many insurance companies are reluctant to provide health or life protection. Availability of members of the health care team and open communication are extremely helpful. However, the possibility of late sequelae such as the development of secondary malignancy may also have to be considered in this context.

Effects of conditioning and transplantation on growth and development of pediatric patients have been discussed above. Health maintenance and early detection of problems are important features, probably for several decades. Denial of past events and the desire to be equal to their peers may result in severe problems with compliance in this age group of patients. An interdisciplinary approach involving adolescent medicine physicians along with endocrinologists, group therapy and peer support groups appears most promising. Rehabilitation should begin at the time of diagnosis and should involve a long term treatment plan.

In 1972 a National Cancer Institute sponsored conference identified four objectives for rehabilitation:

1. Psychological support once cancer has been diagnosed;

2. Optimal physical functioning following cancer treatment;

3. Vocational counseling as early as possible where indicated;

4. Optimal social functioning as the ultimate goal of all cancer control treatment.

The past 15 years have seen a great deal of progress. Progress can be achieved by setting goals that are realistic and consistent with physiological and environmental limitations. Survivors of transplantation may benefit from participation in self-help groups such as National Coalition of Cancer Survivors. Increases in involvement will impact our society in its entirety.

References

Nims JW (1991) Survivorship and rehabilitation. In: Whedon MB (ed), Bone Marrow Transplantation, Principles, Practice and Nursing Insights. Jones & Bartlett, Boston 334–345

Wingard JR, Curbow B, Baker F, Piantadosi S (1991) Health, functional status, and employment of adult survivors of bone marrow transplantation. Ann Intern Med 114:113–118

Outlook

Bone marrow transplantation is a complex procedure. However, the basic purpose is that of transferring normal lymphohemopoietic stem cells for lymphohemopoietic reconstitution, and to supply cells with normal genetic information central to metabolic pathways in the recipient organism. At present these functions are incompletely achieved. Consequently, the future of marrow transplantation will depend upon increasing the efficacy of these functions and lessening associated side effects. Quite likely the next generation of marrow transplantation will be different, in appearance, from the procedures used at the present time. The most important problems still to be mastered are those of recurrence of the underlying disease, prevention of GVHD without jeopardizing engraftment, prevention of infection and prevention of delayed adverse effects.

Preventing recurrence of leukemia, lymphoma or other malignancies will require a more effective eradication of clonogenic tumor cells than is presently possible. Currently employed regimens are of maximum tolerated intensity. This is true for both chemotherapeutic and irradiation approaches. It is possible that combinations of different agents similar to combined modality treatment of lymphohemopoietic malignancies or solid tumors will have improved efficacy in eradicating malignant cells. Assuming that non-marrow toxicity is not prohibitive, marrow infusion used as a rescue procedure should then result in cure of most patients. However, progress in this field has been slow. Experimental studies indicate that coupling of radioisotopes to monoclonal antibodies directed at tumor cells might allow for in situ delivery of high dose radiation without unacceptable damage to organs other than the lymphohemopoietic system. A sufficiently rapid radioactive decay, so as to limit the time period of impaired marrow function prior to marrow infusion, would allow for successful applications of this method. It may also be possible to couple immunotoxins such as ricin chain A to monoclonal antibodies for in vivo or in vitro treatment of remaining tumor cells.

A graft-vs-leukemia effect, long recognized in experimental models, has also been shown to play a role in clinical studies. However, attempts to take advantage of such an effect to reduce the probability of leukemic relapse and improve survival have been frustrating. Data obtained in murine systems suggest that it should be possible to separate a graft-vs-leukemia effect from GVHD, which in turn would allow for reduced recurrence rates without putting the patient at risk of dying from GVHD. It is of interest that a few cases of patients with chronic myelogenous leukemia have been reported who showed a transient cytogenetic relapse (in the form of Philadelphia chromosome positive cells) after transplantation. Subsequently, Philadelphia chromosome positive cells disappeared, and the patients have been followed and found to remain in remission for prolonged periods of time. It is conceivable that the reappearance of these cells might have triggered a leukemia-reactive donor derived cell clone, leading to the elimination of the leukemic cells. Some investigators have expanded this concept and infused patients who had suffered a post-transplant relapse with donor buffy coat cells. Indeed, several patients were induced into remission and are currently surviving without evidence of leukemia. Post-transplantation immunotherapy with interferon, interleukin-1, interleukin-2, alone or in conjunction with lymphokine activated killer (LAK) cells is currently under investigation. In vitro culture of the marrow in the presence of interleukin-2 prior to transplantation has been proposed as an alternative.

Progress has been made in regards to the prevention of GVHD. Regimens using combinations of cyclosporine and methylprednisolone, or cyclosporine and methotrexate, have reduced the incidence of clinically relevant acute GVHD to approximately 15–30% in patients given HLA-identical marrow grafts. Some studies using intravenous immunoglobulin in addition suggest a GVHD incidence of only 10%. The incidence of GVHD is still high in HLA genotypically non-identical marrow grafts from either related or unrelated donors. On the other hand, if a graft-vs-leukemia effect exists, one might speculate that profound immunosuppression might reduce such an effect and result in increased probability of leukemic relapse. Conceivably, shortening the prophylactic immunosuppressive regimen might reduce that risk.

T-cell depletion of marrow by various techniques has been explored widely. However, successful depletion of T-cells by two or three logs or more, albeit successful in preventing GVHD, may also prevent sustained engraftment and result in an increased incidence of leukemia relapse. It has been postulated that less complete depletion, i.e., leaving in place a certain number of T-lymphocytes, might facilitate engraftment and still allow for prevention of GVHD. This, however, is controversial. Alternatively, one could attempt more selective depletion of, e.g., CD4 or CD8 positive T lymphocytes. In fact studies using this approach are underway but results are still preliminary. Alternatively, complete T-cell depletion might be acceptable if other means are found to ensure engraftment. Several monoclonal antibodies directed at class I or II histocompatibility antigens, or at adhesion molecules (e.g., CD44) have been used in murine and canine models, and an antibody directed at the human lymphocyte function antigen (LFA) 1 has been used successfully clinically in facilitating engraftment, even of histoincompatible marrow. Finally, exciting data obtained in murine models show that mice transplanted with a combination of T-cell depleted autologous marrow and unmanipulated histoincompatible allogeneic marrow not only achieved engraftment but also failed to develop GVHD. Concurrent administration of interleukin-2 (early after transplantation) may consolidate this effect and in addition exert an anti-leukemia effect.

Another approach to the prevention of GVHD is the use of autologous marrow. In recent years, autologous marrow transplants have been carried out with increasing frequency and with good success rates for non-Hodgkin lymphomas, Hodgkin disease, or acute non-lymphoblastic leukemias. A major problem, however, is recurrence of the underlying disease. It is not clear whether this is due to proliferation of clonogenic cells surviving the conditioning regimen in the patient or tumor cells present in the marrow and re-infused following conditioning. Although a contribution by re-infused cells is possible, the high recurrence rate in certain patient groups even with allogenenic marrow transplantation suggests that the most important problem is that of relative inefficacy of the conditioning regimen. In agreement with this concept, some investigators point out that there is no significant difference in relapse rate between patients given autologous purged or unpurged marrow. In any event, as far as eradication of tumor cells in the patients is concerned, approaches similar to those being tried for allogeneic transplants might be useful. Some investigators have cultured autologous marrow from patients with leukemia in vitro with the goal of eradicating leukemic cells. Preliminary data suggest that this is indeed possible. However, it remains to be seen whether this approach is truly useful clinically.

As an alternative to autologous marrow, autologous peripheral blood could be used as a source of stem cells. Increased numbers of committed precursor cells can be obtained during a rebound phase following treatment of patients with cytotoxic agents or after stimulation with recombinant growth factors (e.g., G-CSF, GM-CSF). The feasibility of this approach was initially shown in animals, and recent clinical data in small numbers of patients suggest successful hemopoietic reconstitution.

An ambitious goal has been the positive selection of hemopoietic stem cells from marrow or peripheral blood. Experimental data in mice, monkeys and more recently in man indicate that such an approach is feasible for autologous transplantation. There is concern, however, that transplantation of purified stem cells may be problematic in the allogeneic setting due to difficulties with engraftment as described for T-cell depleted marrow (IV.3). Conceivably accessory cells facilitating engraftment of stem cells need to be infused concurrently. Alternatively, one could attempt to manipulate the stroma or microenvironment in the recipient in which stem cells are expected to settle. A lead in that direction may have been provided by the in vivo use of monoclonal antibodies in animals and man. We are currently developing a better understanding of the homing behavior of lymphoid and hemopoietic cell populations. Once the responsible receptors have been recognized, manipulations could preferentially lodge stem cells in predetermined sites, such as the marrow cavity.

For numerous indications, autologous stem cells clearly offer an alternative to allogeneic marrow transplantation. In other diseases, for example, congenital disorders, autologous stem cells, if available, would not be useful since the original disease would be re-introduced. Since not all patients have a suitable allogeneic donor, it would be desirable to expand the donor pool by recruiting unrelated volunteer donors or by using cadaveric marrow. A national donor bank for volunteer marrow donors (National Marrow Donor Program) is currently being established in the United States and similar organizations exist in the United Kingdom, Canada, Germany and France. Several hundred successful transplants from unrelated volunteer donors have been reported already; however, only patients with a commonly occurring HLA haplotype, are likely to find donors quickly. Also, it has become apparent that numerous problems, e.g., GVHD and immunoreconstitution, are more formidable after unrelated than after related donor transplants. Additional work is necessary to improve GVHD prevention and immunoreconstitution.

With the use of recombinant DNA technology quantities of hemopoietic growth factors sufficient for clinical studies have become available. G-CSF, GM-CSF, interleukin-3, c-kit ligand, and others have been used already. G-CSF and GM-CSF have yielded encouraging results in regards to hemopoietic reconstitution after transplantation. Conceivably, the use of these factors may facilitate engraftment of T cell-depleted and stem cell-enriched fractions of allogeneic marrow.

One of the most exciting areas of current research is that of gene manipulation or gene transfer into various cell populations including stem cells. Numerous problems in particular of gene expression still exist. Currently the most widely used approach is that involving helper-free retroviral vectors in conjunction with co-culture systems. In mice, monkeys or dogs, the expression of transfected genes for years following the procedure has now been documented. At least two human patients with adenosine deaminase (ADA) deficiency have been treated with autologous lymphocytes into which a normal ADA gene had been inserted. These patients have shown unequivocal improvement of their cellular immune functions. The transfer of normal genetic information into autologous cells with defective or (or absent) information for the respective enzyme or molecule would be the treatment of choice for numerous congenital disorders such as immune deficiencies or storage diseases. As it stands, however, additional work is needed to assure appropriate and sustained gene regulation and expression.

Finally, considering the large numbers of patients that are given solid organ grafts such as kidney, liver, heart, heart/lung and pancreas, generally requiring immunosuppressive treatment with all the associated risks for their entire life, it would be desirable to develop methods to provide an organ transplant recipient with an immune system that would accept the transplanted organ indefinitely without requiring continued immunosuppression. The transfer of lymphohemopoietic cells containing appropriate donor histocompability genes prior to the actual organ transplant would be such an approach.

In summary, present and future work in the field of marrow transplantation will aim at more effective eradication of malignant cells, stem cell enrichment, improved allogeneic engraftment, abrogation of resistance to manipulated grafts and accelerated immunoreconstitution along with graft tolerance. Molecular biology technology is aimed at developing methods which allow for consistent expression of transfected genes in stem cells and other cell populations and together with actual transplant efforts, allow for preferential survival of the transfected cells in the recipient.

References

Andrews RG, Singer JW, Bernstein ID (1990) Human hematopoietic precursors in long term culture: single CD34+ cells that lack detectable T, B, and myeloid antigens produce multiple colony-forming cells when cultured with marrow stromal cells. J Exp Med 172:355–358

Appelbaum FR (1989) The clinical use of hematopoietic growth factors. Semin Hematol 26:7–14

Badger CC, Bernstein ID (1989) Treatment of murine lymphoma with anti-thy 1.1 antibodies. In: Reif AE, Schlesinger M (eds), Thy-1: Immunology, Neurology, and Therapeutic Applications. Marcel Dekker, New York 515–529

Berenson RJ, Andrews RG, Bensinger WI, Kalamasz D, Knitter G, Buckner CD, Bernstein ID (1988) Antigen CD34$^+$ marrow cells engraft lethally irradiated baboons. J Clin Invest 81:951–955

Culver K, Cornetta K, Morgan R, Morecki S, Aebersold P, Kasid A, Lotze M, Rosenberg SA, Anderson WF, Blaese RM (1991) Lymphocytes as cellular vehicles for gene therapy in mouse and man. Proc Natl Acad Sci USA 88:3155–3159

Gribben JG, Freedman AS, Neuberg D, Roy DC, Blake KW, Woo SD, Grossbard ML, Rabinowe SN, Coral F, Freeman GJ, Ritz J, Nadler LM (1991) Immunologic purging of marrow assessed by PCR before autologous bone marrow transplantation for B-cell lymphoma. N Engl J Med 325:1525–1533

Hardy CL, Matsuoka T, Tavassoli M (1991) Distribution of homing protein on hemopoietic stromal and progenitor cells. Exp Hematol 19:968–972

Jalkanen S, Reichert RA, Gallatin WM, Bargatze RF, Weissman IL, Butcher EC (1986) Homing receptors and the control of lymphocyte migration. Immunol Rev 91:39–60

Miller AD (1990) Progress toward human gene therapy. Blood 76:271–278

Rosenberg SA, Aebersold P, Cornetta K, Kasid A, Morgan RA, Moen R, Karson EM, Lotze MT, Yang JC, Topalian SL, Merino MJ, Culver K, Miller AD, Blaese RM, Anderson WF (1990) Gene transfer into humans – immunotherapy of patients with advanced melanoma, using tumor-infiltrating lymphocytes modified by retroviral gene transduction. N Engl J Med 323:570–578

Spangrude GJ, Heimfeld S, Weissman IL (1988) Purification and characterization of mouse hematopoietic stem cells. Science 241:58–62

Sykes M, Romick ML, Hoyles KA, Sachs DH (1990) In vivo administration of interleukin 2 plus T cell-depleted syngeneic marrow prevents graft-versus-host disease mortality and permits alloengraftment. J Exp Med 171:645–658

Truitt RL, LeFever AV, Shih CCY, Jeske HM, Martin TM (1990) Graft-versus-leukemia effect. In: Burakoff SJ, Deeg HJ, Ferrara J, Atkinston K. (eds), Graft-versus-host disease: immunology, pathophysiology, and treatment. Marcel Dekker, New York 177–204

Thomas ED (1990) Bone marrow transplantation – past, present and future. In: The Nobel Prizes. Stockholm, Sweden: The Nobel Foundation

Glossary

Allogeneic: From a different individual of the same species.

Autologous (= autochthonous): From the same individual; in marrow transplantation this means from the same patient.

Bone Marrow Transplantation: The intravenous infusion of marrow cells obtained by multiple aspirates from the bones (usually the posterior iliac crests) of the donor, into the recipient (patient, host). The relevant marrow cells (stem cells) find their way to the bone by a mechanism termed "homing" (via the nutritional arteries), settle in "niches" and begin to replicate and repopulate the patient's marrow cavities and blood.

Chimera: An individual who hosts (indefinitely) cells of different genetic origin. In a marrow chimera, the donor-derived cells repopulate the patient's hemopoietic and immune system. For example, if a transplant is carried out from a female donor into a male patient and the transplant is successful, the patient will have female lymphohemopoietic cells for the rest of his life.

Conditioning: The preparation of the patient for marrow transplantation. Conditioning is aimed at eradicating the patient's own cells (malignant cells of the disease for which treatment is being given, and immuno-competent cells of the patient's immune system) to allow for engraftment of donor cells. Conditioning may include the use of gamma irradiation, cytotoxic and immunosuppressive drugs, monoclonal or polyclonal antibodies, and in the near future, possibly radioisotopes and immunotoxins.

Donor: The individual from whom the marrow cells (or blood cells used for transfusions) are obtained.

Engraftment: About 2–3 weeks after infusion of bone marrow, granulocytes (in the case of allogeneic transplantation of donor origin) appear in the peripheral blood indicating that donor cells have begun to replicate, i.e., the transplant has engrafted. Engraftment can also be demonstrated by bone marrow biopsy which shows granulocyte, red blood cell, and platelet precursors, usually around day 14.

Graft-Versus-Host Disease (GVHD): Presumably all transplants other than autologous or syngeneic result in a graft-versus-host reaction, i.e., an interaction between donor-derived and host cells. If a state of tolerance develops, there may be no manifestations of this interaction. In many instances, however, this interaction may result in tissue damage especially to skin, intestinal tract and liver, and lead to clinical dysfunction of those organs, termed GVHD. This reaction is triggered by donor-derived T cells.

HLA: Abbreviation for "Human Leukocyte Antigens". These antigens were found originally on leukocytes, especially lymphocytes, but some of them (HLA class I antigens) are expressed widely and possibly on all nucleated cells. The genetic information that is responsible for the expression of these antigens is located on the short arm of chromosome 6 in a region called the major histocompatibility complex. Within this complex, dependent upon structure and function, three classes (I, II and III) of antigens are differentiated. Class I antigens are defined biochemically as dimers of a glycoprotein of 45 Kd molecular weight, linked noncovalently to beta 2-microglobulin. Class II antigens are defined biochemically as glycoprotein dimers of approximately 29 and 34 Kd molecular weight respectively. These HLA antigens play a central role in the interaction of immunocompetent cells, and in the interaction between donor and host cells. They are also responsible for mutual recognition of cells in mixed leukocyte culture. Class III antigens represent complement components and some other factors.

Host: The recipient of a transplant (of marrow or a solid organ), i.e., the patient.

Host-Versus-Graft Reaction: A function of host cells with a detrimental effect on donor cells. If the host-versus-graft reaction is stronger than the graft-versus-host reaction, it will result in rejection (or non-acceptance) of the graft, i.e., the graft fails (does not take).

Mismatch: If host and donor HLA type (A, B, D/DR) are not genotypically identical, a mismatch situation exists. This includes the rare case of phenotypic identity, where the various antigens appear to be the same in donor and host but family studies show that they are derived from a different genetic background. If one, two or three antigens are phenotypically different we refer to a one, two or three antigen (one haplotype) mismatch. As techniques of molecular biology have become available, the degree of matching or mismatching is being determined more and more at the molecular level (isoelectric focusing, restriction fragment length polymorphism (RFLP), site specific oligonucleotide probes (SSOP).

Mixed Lymphocyte Culture (MLC): Lymphocytes of patient and donor are co-cultured for 6 days in tissue culture plates. Usually one cell population is inactivated by irradiation or mitomycin. If lymphocytes of patient and donor differ at the HLA D/DR region, the non-inactivated population will proliferate. The amount of proliferation, measured by thymidine incorporation, can be used as a relative measure of histoincompatibility between donor and patient.

Non-HLA Antigens: Histocompatibility antigens other than HLA, also called minor antigens, encoded for by genes outside the major histocompatibility complex and often on different chromosomes. In man, these antigens are poorly defined.

Syngeneic: From a different but genetically identical individual, i.e., from a monozygotic twin.

Xenogeneic: From an individual of a different species.

Subject Index

ABO-incompatible marrow
 transplant 58, 233
abortion 266
acquired immunodeficiency syndrome (AIDS) 25, 38, 171
acrolein 111
acute lymphoblastic leukemia (see
 also ALL) 8, 18–20
acute myeloblastic leukemia (see also
 AML) 16, 17
acyclovir 161, 178, 183, 208, 219,
 231
– high dose 161
– – oral 171
– – systemic 171
adenovirus 168, 182, 211, 284
adrenal gland 264
aerobic bacteria, selective depletion 160
age related toxicity 9, 14, 17
agglutination, soybean 134
ALL (acute lymphoblastic
 leukemia) 8, 18
– age 19
– cytogenetic abnormality 19
– immunophenotype 19
– relapse 20
– – CNS 20
– – testicular 20
– therapy
– – non-transplant 8
– – transplantation 8
allergy 52
allogeneic transplant/transplanta-
 tion 9, 24, 56, 121
allosensitization 12, 13, 121, 141,
 142

– of the donor 7, 38, 39
alopecia 114
aminoglycoside 163, 207
AML (acute myeloblastic
 leukemia) 16
– cytogenetic abnormality 18
– disease-free survival 17
– early relapse 17
– first remission 17
– transplant 18
– – autologous 18
– – unrelated 18
amphotericin B 164
– low dose 160
– nebulized 161
– nephrotoxicity 165
anemia
– aplastic 1, 13, 39, 133, 142, 144,
 177, 275
– – untransfused 13
– microangiopathic hemolytic
 (MAHA) 211, 218
– refractory (RA) 16
– – with excess blasts (RAEB)
 16
– – with excess blasts in transformation (RAEBT) 16
anesthetic risk 38
Anthony Nolan Appeal 33
anti-endotoxin monoclonal antibody 166
antibiotic
– non-resorbable 160
– prophylactic oral coverage
 170
antibody
– lymphocytotoxic 39

antibody (cont.)
- monoclonal   129, 132, 137, 146, 148, 275
-- humanized   137
-- anti-endotoxin   166
antiemetics   110
antigen, histocompatibility   1
antigen-presenting cell   123
antigenic peptide   123
antithymocyte globulin (see ATG)
aplasia, marrow   1
aplastic anemia   1, 13, 39, 133, 142, 144, 177, 275
- untransfused   13
Ara C (cytosine arabinoside)   217
aseptic necrosis   137, 279, 283
aspergillosis, pulmonary   158
Aspergillus   220
ATG (antithymocyte globulin)   13, 130, 143, 146, 275
autologous transplant/transplantation   9, 23, 24, 33, 57, 149, 276, 289
- versus allgeneic   54
- autoplantation   34
azathioprine   201
azoospermia   266

B-cell cancer   171
- pleomorphic lymphoma   275
back-up marrow   97
BACT variant   80
bacteremia   158
bare lymphocyte syndrome   10
BCNU   116
biomagnetic sphere   112, 148
biopsy, open lung   169, 175, 181
bladder irrigation   112
blood
- culture   163
- gas   175
body image   283
bone age   265
breast carcinoma   24, 62
bronchiolitis, obliterative   185
bronchoalveolar lavage   169, 175, 179

bronchoscopy   169
busulfan   22, 193, 217, 270, 280
- plus cyclophosphamide   79

cadaveric marrow   100
Campath 1   133
Candida   221
- krusei   160
candidiasis, hepatosplenic   158
capillary leak syndrome   117, 205
capital alopecia   114
capsule, posterior   269
cardiotoxicity   115
carmustine (BCNU)   116
cataract   269
"catastrophic illness"   61
catheter, indwelling   159, 165
- care of   159
- removal   165
catheterization   112
CBV   80
CD4+ T-cells   124
CD8+ T-cells   124
CD44   146
ceftazidime   163
cell
- antigen-presenting   123
- dendritic   145
- LAK   135
- natural killer   124
- purging   34
- stem   2, 98, 150, 287
-- peripheral blood   16, 23, 35, 150, 290
- stromal   152
- T-lymphocyte/cell (see also T-lymphocyte)   2, 9, 12, 37, 95, 121, 123-125, 132, 146, 147, 275, 289
cerebellar toxicity   114
chemoprophylaxis   159
chemoradiotherapy regimen   75
chemoseparation   134
chemotherapy regimen   78
chest
- radiography   175, 229
-- routine   163

Subject Index

– radiotherapy 178
chicken pox 231
"chimera" 2
– "mixed" 142
chromosomal marker 233
chronic
– granulomatous disease 10
– lymphocytic leukemia 34
– myelogenous leukemia (see also CML) 21, 22
– myelomonocytic leukemia (CMML) 16
ciprofloxacin 160
clonal
– deletion 125
– evolution 12, 275
– expansion 123
– hemopoiesis 16
Clostridium difficile 166
CML (chronic myelogenous leukemia) 21
– autologous transplantation 22
– blast transformation 21
– phase
– – accelerated 21
– – chronic 21
CMML (chronic myelomonocytic leukemia) 16
CMV (cytomegalovirus) 38, 152, 175, 198
– blood products
– – negative 168, 184
– – positive 178
– interstitial pneumonitis 178
– – prophylaxis 168
CNS involvement 19
co-morbid medical problem 51
co-trimoxazole 160
cognitive function 280
combined immunodeficiency 10
– severe (see also SCID) 9, 10, 37, 133
common site of infection 159
complement 148
compliance 283
complications, delayed 230

conditioning regimen 11, 283
– approaches to improving 83, 84
– current use 75
– function 67
– future developments 86
– oral hygiene 107
– regimen-related toxicity 125, 149
– – schema 106
– requirement 70
– side effects 105
– second transplant 83
confirmation of diagnosis 49
congenital disease 9
conjunctivae 269
consultation 25
– referral and initial 43
cornea, perforation 270
corneal stippling 270
cost, transplantation 61
cost-benefit ratio 62
counter flow elutriation 134
cranial irradiation 20, 264, 270, 280
crossover 35
cryopreservation 94, 150
Cryptococcus 221
cutaneous toxicity 114
cyclophosphamide 2, 11, 78, 114, 115, 129, 143, 209, 266, 280
– plus TBI (total body irradiation) 75, 76
– plus TLI (total lymphoid irradiation) 76
cyclosporine 2, 13, 125, 129, 137, 177, 188, 200, 207, 208, 218, 233, 265, 275, 280
cystitis, hemorrhagic 112, 205, 209, 211, 280
cytarabine, with/without cyclophosphamide plus TBI (total body irradiation) 77
cytogenetic analysis 149
cytomegalovirus (see also CMV) 38, 152, 168, 175, 178, 184, 198
cytoreduction, pre-conditioning 80
cytosine arabinoside (Ara C) 217

debility, persistent 47
decontamination 136
deletion, clonal 125
dendritic cell 145
dental development 279
depletion
– leukocyte 145
– – T-lymphocyte/cell 2, 9, 12, 37, 95, 121, 132, 146, 147, 275, 289
– plasma 95
– red cell 95
– selective 289
– – aerobic bacteria 160
depression 283
dermatitis, radiation recall 114
desoxycortisol 264
development 20
– dental 279
– sexual 265
dexamethasone 110
diagnosis, confirmation 49
dialysis 113
diarrhea 111
– infectious 166
diphenhydramine 110
discussion
– with the patient 46
– with the potential donor 48
disease
– recurrence 233, 283
– status 50
– underlying 72
divorce 284
DMSO 98
donor
– age 38, 39
– allosensitization 7, 38, 39
– anesthetic risk 38
– consideration 156
– haploidentical 9
– HLA (human leukocyte antigen)-identical 10
– leukemic cells 234, 273
– normal 55
– preference 54
– pregnancy test 38

– psychological stability 38
– related, (family) 31
– unrelated 9, 14, 18, 31, 63, 291
dopamine 165

EBV (Epstein-Barr virus) 171, 275
ectropion 270
electrolyte imbalance 117
emesis 110
encephalopathy 213
endotracheal intubation 179
engraftment
– facilitating 289, 290
– marker of 57
– sustained 14
– – failure of 3, 12, 37, 39, 121, 132, 133, 141, 145, 148, 151, 233
Epstein-Barr virus (EBV) 171, 275
erythrocyte, support 58
etoposide, with/without cyclophosphamide plus TBI (total body irradiation) 77
evaluation
– histocompatibility 56
– medical 49

failure, of sustained engraftment 3, 12, 37, 39, 121, 132, 133, 141, 145, 148, 151, 233
family donor 31
Fanconi anemia 12
fertility 266
fetal liver cell transplantation 9
fever 159
FK506 137, 252
flowers 159
fluconazole 160
fluid
– imbalance 117
– overload 182
food
– intake 232
– low-bacterial content 159
foscarnet 161

fungal infection, deep   158

G-CSF (granulocyte colony-stimulating factor)   162
ganciclovir   161, 168, 178, 183, 184, 198, 209, 219
gastroenteritis   111
Gaucher disease   11
gene transfer   34, 291
genotypic identity   36
germ cell tumor   24
German measles   231
germfree environment   135
globulin, antithymocyte (ATG)   13, 130, 143, 146, 275
glucocorticoid   265
GM-CSF (granulocyte-macrophage colony-stimulating factor)   162
Gnotobiosis   135
graft
– composition   72
– failure   3, 12, 37, 39, 121, 132, 133, 141, 145, 148, 151, 233
– rejection   13, 34, 39
graft-versus-host disease (secondary disease, see GVHD)
graft-versus-host reaction   121, 149
graft-versus-leukemia effect   34, 130, 135, 254, 288
granulomatous disease, chronic   10
growth
– and development   20
– factor, hemopoietic   13, 35, 62, 151, 162, 167, 290, 291
– hormone   264
– spurt   264
– velocity   264
GVHD (graft-versus-host disease/secondary disease)   2, 34, 37, 39, 95, 121, 146, 191, 211, 283
– acute   121, 194
– afferent phase   123
– autologous   122
– chronic   124, 195, 231, 233, 237, 263, 273
– – management of infections   170

– – prognosis   249
– efferent arm   124
– HLA (human leukocyte antigen)-nonidentical transplant   131
– morbidity   131
– mortality   128
– probability   147
– prophylaxis   2, 147
– risk   143
– syngeneic   122, 125
– transfusion-induced   233
– treatment   136

hand washing   231
haploidentical donor   9
haplotype   35, 36
harvest procedure   89
HBV (hepatitis B)   197
HCV (hepatitis C)   197
health maintenance   284
hemopoietic growth factor   13, 35, 62, 151, 162, 167, 290, 291
hemoglobinuria, paroxysmal nocturnal   13, 15
hemolytic uremic syndrome (HUS)   113, 233, 280
hemopoiesis, clonal   16
hemorrhagic
– cystitis   112, 205, 209, 211, 280
– myocarditis   115
HEPA (high-efficiency particulate air) filtration   159, 160
hepatic damage   113, 114
– drug-induced   200
hepatitis virus   38
– hepatitis B (HBV)   197
– hepatitis C (HCV)   197
hepatosplenic candidiasis   158
herpes simplex virus (see also HSV)   161, 168, 182, 198, 222
high grade histology   22
high-efficiency particulate air (HEPA) filtration   159, 160
Hiroshima   1
hirsutism   283

Subject Index

histocompatibility 35
- antigen 1
- evaluation 56
histoincompatible transplant 145
HIV (human immunodeficiency virus) 25, 38, 171
HLA (human leukocyte antigen)
- haplotypes 14
- identical 10
- incompatible 12
- nonidentical 37, 275
- typing 17
Hodgkin disease 22, 23
- marrow involvement 23
homing 291
hormone replacement 266
host 141, 274
- milieu 274
- response 141
HSV (herpes simplex virus) 168, 182, 198, 222
- reactivation 161
- resistance to acyclovir 161
human immunodeficiency virus (HIV) 25, 38, 171
Hurler disease 11
HUS (hemolytic uremic syndrome) 113, 233, 280
hydroxyurea 22
hyperhydration 112
hyperplasia, nodular regenerative (NRH) 191
hyperthyroidism 263
hypogonadism, primary 265
hypothyroidism 263
hypoxemia 179, 231

imbalance, fluid and electrolyte 117
immediate post-transplant phase 158
immunization, re-immunization 170
immunodeficiency 246
- aquired immunodeficiency syndrome (AIDS) 25, 38, 171
- combined 10
- - severe (see also SCID) 9, 10, 37, 133

immunoglobulin
- intravenous 131, 183, 288
- preparation 161
immunoprophylaxis 159, 161
immunoreconstitution 291
immunosuppression 14, 70
- degree of 71
immunotoxin 134, 148, 288
- conjugate 133
inclusion body 181
indication of transplantation 7
indwelling catheter 159, 165
- care of 159
- removal 165
infection 137, 230
- common site 159
- mortality 10
- potential 52
- pre-transplant 57
- principles of management 156
- prophylaxis 159
- signs 162
- unresolved 157
initial
- consultation 43
- discussion 46
insurance
- carrier 61
- coverage 26
interdisciplinary approach 284
interferon 21
interleukin-1 123
interleukin-2 123, 135, 288
intermediate post-transplant phase 167
interstitial pneumonitis 22, 116, 168, 175
- CMV (cytomegalovirus) 175
- GVHD 177
- idiopathic 175, 177
- - mortality 183
- incidence 177
- risk factors 176
- therapy 116
intraocular lens 270
intubation, endotracheal 179
irradiation 1

- cranial 20, 264, 270, 280
- mediastinal 22
- syndromes 1
- total body (see also TBI) 1, 144, 177, 178, 184, 264, 269, 273
- thoracoabdominal 12, 144, 276
- total lymphoid (TLI) 144, 273
- UV light 144
isotope, radioactive 133, 287

joint replacement 279

lacrimal gland 269
LAK cell 135
late post-transplant phase 170
lens, intraocular 270
leukemia
- acute lymphoblastic (see also ALL) 8, 18–20
- acute myeloblastic (see also AML) 16–18
- chronic lymphocytic 34
- chronic myelogenous (see also CML) 21, 22
- chronic myelomonocytic (CMML) 16
- donor cells 234, 273
- relapse 17, 135, 289
leukocyte
- adhesion defect 10
- depletion 145
- filter 178
- peripheral blood 143
leukoencephalopathy 20, 213, 214, 216
LFA I (lymphocyte function antigen I) 146
longterm survivor 14
lung, open biopsy 169, 175, 181
lymphoblastic leukemia, acute (see also ALL) 8, 18–20
lymphocyte
- large granular 124
- T-cell (see T-lymphocyte)
lymphocytic leukemia, chronic 34
lymphocytotoxic antibody 39
lymphohemopoietic malignancy 177

lymphoid irradiation, total (TLI) 144, 273
lymphoma 22, 34, 275
- lymphoblastic 22
- non-Hodgkin 22, 34
- pleomorphic B-cell 275
lymphoproliferative disorder 273

M-CSF (macrophage colony-stimulating factor) 165
magnetic biosphere 134
MAHA (microangiopathic hemolytic anemia) 211, 218
malignancy
- lymphohemopoietic 177
- secondary 12, 144, 273
marital dysfunction 284
marker of engraftment 57
marrow
- ABO-incompatible 58, 233
- aplasia 1
- autologous 23, 33, 289
- back-up 97
- cadaveric 100
- fibrosis 16
- harvest 89
- purging 19, 150, 290
- source 31, 32
- storage 93
- transplantation (see transplant/transplantation)
MDS (myelodyplastic syndrome) 16
measles 231
- German 231
mediastinal
- irradiation 22
- mass 19
medical evaluation 49
melanoma 24
menopause 267
mesna 112
metabolic storage diseases 10
methotrexate 2, 20, 129, 177, 201, 214, 273
methylprednisolone 137, 273
metoclopramide 110
metronidozole 166

Subject Index

microangiopathic hemolytic anemia (MAHA) 211, 218
microenvironment 141, 152, 290
"mixed chimera" 142
MLC (mixed leukocyte culture) 36
monoclonal antibody 129, 132, 137, 146, 148, 275
- anti-endotoxin 166
- humanized 137
monotherapy 163
monozygotic (syngeneic) twin 2, 31, 121, 122
- transplant 177
morbidity 26
mortality 26
mucositis 107
- therapy 110
muscle wasting 284
myeloblastic leukemia, acute (see also AML) 16–18
myelodyplastic syndrome (MDS) 16
myelodysplasia 13
myelogenous leukemia, chronic (see also CML) 21, 22
myeloma, multiple 24
myelomonocytic leukemia, chronic (CMML) 16
myelosupression 1, 233
myocarditis, hemorrhagic 115

Nagasaki 1
naso-lacrimal duct 270
National Marrow Donor Program 33
natural killer cell 124
nausea 110
necrosis, aseptic 137, 279, 283
nephrotoxicity 112, 207
neuroblastoma 25
neuropathy, peripheral 115
neuropsychological deficit 280
neurotoxicity 114
neutrophil transfusion 161, 166
- prophylactic 161
- therapeutic 166
nodular regenerative hyperplasia (NRH) 191

non-Hodgkin lymphoma 22, 34
non-marrow toxicity 287
nutrition, parenteral 187, 201

oncogene 274
open lung biopsy 169, 175, 181
opsonization 132
oral
- hygiene regimen 107
- prophylactic antibiotic coverage 170
organ transplantation 122
osteoporosis 267, 283
ototoxicity 115
ovarian function 265, 266

pancreatitis 137
parenteral nutrition 187, 201
paroxysmal nocturnal hemoglobinuria 13, 15
patient
- consideration 157
- nontransplant 276
- untransfused 143, 144
penicillin, antipseudomonal 163
pentoxifylline 165, 184, 193
peptide, antigenic 123
perforation of the cornea 270
peripheral blood
- leukocyte 143
- stem cell 16, 23, 150, 290
- - mobilisation 35
peripheral neuropathy 115
persistent debility 47
phenotypic identity 32, 36, 145
Philadelphia chromosome 19, 20, 288
physical measures 159
plants 159
plasma depletion 95
plasmapheresis 39
platelet transfusion 233
pleomorphic B-cell lymphoma 275
Pneumocystis 175
- carinii 168, 182, 253

pneumonitis, interstitial (see also interstitial pneumonitis) 22, 116, 168, 175–177, 183
polyomavirus 211
post-transplant/transplantation
– phase 158, 167, 170
– – immediate 158
– – intermediate 167
– – late 170
– therapy 82
pox, chicken 231
pre-conditioning cytoreduction 80
pre-transplant/transplantation
– management of infection 57
– phase (before day 0) 157
prednisone 130
preference of donor 54
pregnancy 266
– test 38
preparation for marrow transplantation 43
previous treatment 51
prophylaxis
– infections 159
– neutrophil transfusion 161
– oral antibiotic coverage 170
– urotoxicity 112
prostaglandin 179
– instillation 112
psychological
– assessment 53
– stability 38
– stress 26, 63
pulmonary
– aspergillosis 158
– non-infectious complications 168
purging
– cells 34
– marrow 19, 150, 290
– tumor cells 96
PUVA (psoralen and ultraviolet irradiation) 129, 252

RA (refractory anemia) 16
radiation
– accident 25

– recall dermatitis 114
radioactive isotope 133, 287
radiography
– chest 175, 229
– – routine 163
– facial sinuses, routine 163
radioimmunopharmaceutical 82
radiotherapy, chest 178
RAEB (refractory anemia with excess blasts) 16
RAEBT (refractory anemia with excess blasts in transformation) 16
re-immunization 170
receptor, T-cell 123
red cell depletion 95
referral consultation 43
referring physician, role of 45
refractory anemia (RA) 16
– with excess blasts (RAEB) 16
– with excess blasts in transformation (RAEBT) 16
regimen-related toxicity 125, 149
– schema 106
rehabilitation 229, 283
rejection 13, 34, 39
relapse 23
– "resistant" 23
– "sensitive" 23
remission, unmaintained 17
renal
– dose 165
– failure 205
– toxicity 112
resistance 141, 145, 148
respiratory distress syndrome, acute 183
respiratory syncytial virus 168
retinopathy 270
retroviral vector 291
RFLP (restriction fragment length polymorphism) 36
rosette formation 134

salivary secretion 232
Schirmer's test 243, 248

Subject Index

SCID (severe combined immunodeficiency) 9, 37, 133
- with ADA deficiency 10
secondary disease (see GVHD, graft-versus-host disease)
secondary malignancy 12, 144, 273
segregation 36
sensitization 72
sequence specific oligonucleotide probe (SSOP) 37
serotonin antagonists 110
severe combined immunodeficiency (see also SCID) 9, 10, 37, 133
sexual/sexuality 284
- activity 232
- development 265
shortness of breath 179
sicca syndrome 270
sickle-cell disease 13
skin contracture 284
source of marrow 31, 32
soybean agglutination 134
sperm production 267
spleen 2
- shielding 2
- transplant 2
- cells 2
splenectomy 22
splenomegaly 22
SSOP (sequence specific oligobucleotide probe) 37
stem cell 150, 287
- peripheral blood 16, 23, 150, 290
- - mobilization 35
- transplant/transplantation 2, 98
stress, psychological 26, 63
stromal cell 152
sun blocking cream 232
"superantigen" 135
survivor, longterm 14
swimming 232
syndrome
- acute respiratory distress 183

- AIDS (aquired immunodeficiency syndrome) 25, 38, 171
- bare lymphocyte 10
- capillary leak 117, 205
- graft-versus-host disease (secondary disease, see also GVHD) 2, 34, 37, 39, 95, 121–125, 128, 131, 136, 143, 146, 147, 170, 191, 194, 195, 211, 233, 237, 249, 263, 273, 283
- Hodgkin 22, 23
- - marrow involvement 23
- Hurler 11
- HUS (hemolytic uremic) 113, 233, 280
- irradiation 1
- myelodyplastic (MDS) 16
- non-Hodgkin 22, 34
- sicca syndrome of the eyes 270
- VOD (veno-occlusive disease) 113, 126, 187, 189, 190, 192, 205–207
- - liver 182
- Wiscott-Aldrich 10
syngeneic (monozygotic) twin 2, 31, 121, 122
- transplant 177

T-lymphocyte/cell 2
- autoreactive 125
- CD4+ T-cell 124
- CD8+ T-cell 124
- depletion 2, 9, 12, 37, 95, 121, 132, 146, 147, 275, 289
- receptor 123
TBI (total body irradiation) 1, 144, 273
- exposure rate 178
- fractionated 177, 184, 264, 269
- single dose 264, 269
tear production 269
teicoplanin 164
test, Schirmer's 243, 248
thalassemia 12
thalidomide 137
therapeutic
- measures 162

- neutrophil transfusion 166
therapy
- discontinuance 164
- empiric 163
- immunosuppressive 14
- monotherapy 163
- post-transplantation 82
- specific 169
thoracoabdominal irradiation 12, 144, 276
thymus 125
thyroid dysfunction 263
timing of transplantation 7, 9
TLI (total lymphoid irradiation) 144, 273
tolerance 124
total
- body irradiation (see also TBI) 1, 144, 177, 178, 184, 264, 269
- lymphoid irradiation (TLI) 144, 273
- protective environment 159
toxicity
- age related 9, 14, 17
- bladder 111
- cardiac 115
- cerebellar 114
- cutaneous 114
- hepatic 113
- marrow transplantation, immediate and delayed 47
- non-marrow 287
- pulmonary 116
- regimen-related 125, 149
- renal 112
- screening 52
- transplant-related 9, 11
Toxoplasma gondii 169, 223
transfusion 10, 53, 122
- GVHD inducing 233
- neutrophil
- - prophylactic 161
- - therapeutic 166
- platelet 233
- prophylactic neutrophil 161
- support 12, 57

- therapeutic neutrophil 166
4:11 translocation 20
transplant/transplantation
- ABO incompatible 58, 233
- allogeneic 9, 24, 54, 56, 121
- autologous 9, 23, 24, 33, 54, 57, 149, 276, 289
- cost 61
- delayed complications 230
- fetal liver cell 9
- histoincompatible 145
- indication 7, 61
- marrow preparation 43
- role of team 43
- second 83, 149
- solid organ 122
- spleen 2
- - cells 2
- stem cells 2, 98
- syngeneic 177
- timing 7, 9
- toxicity, immediate and delayed 47
- transplant-related toxicity 9, 11
treatment, previous 51
trimethoprim-sulfamethoxazole 168, 175, 183
- intolerance 169
tumor
- cell purging 96
- necrosis factor α 124, 136, 179
- solid 24, 273, 275
twin, monozygotic (syngeneic) 2, 31, 121, 122

umbilical cord blood 12
- cells 100
underlying disease 72
unrelated donor 9, 14, 18, 31, 63, 291
untransfused 143, 144
urotoxicity 111
- prophylaxis 112
UV irradiation 144

vaginal dysfunction 232
vaginitis 267, 280

vancomycin 163, 166
varicella zoster virus (VZV) 170, 182, 198, 222, 231
- zoster immune globulin (ZIG) 231
veno-occlusive disease (VOD) 113, 126, 187, 189, 190, 192, 205–207
- liver 182
virus
- adenovirus 168, 182, 211, 284
- cytomegalovirus 38, 152, 168, 175, 178, 184, 198
- Epstein-Barr (EBV) 171, 275
- hepatitis 38
-- HBV (hepatitis B) 197
-- HCV (hepatitis C) 197
- herpes simplex (see also HSV) 161, 168, 182, 198, 222
- human immunodeficiency (HIV) 25, 38, 171
- polyomavirus 211
- respiratory syncytial 168
- varizella zoster (VZV) 170, 182, 198, 222, 231
-- zoster immune globulin (ZIG) 231
VOD (veno-occlusive disease) 113, 126, 187, 189, 190, 192, 205–207
- liver 182
VZV (see varicella zoster virus)

Wiscott-Aldrich syndrome 10

ZIG (zoster immune globulin) 231